Primer of
Sectional Anatomy with MRI and CT Correlation

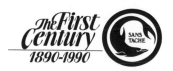

Primer of
Sectional Anatomy with MRI and CT Correlation

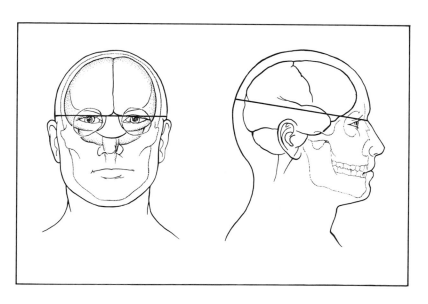

Charles P. Barrett, Ph.D.

Associate Professor of Anatomy
University of Maryland School of Medicine
Baltimore, Maryland

Steven J. Poliakoff, M.D.

Assistant Professor of Anatomy
University of Maryland School of Medicine
Baltimore, Maryland

Lawrence E. Holder, M.D., F.A.C.R.

Director
Department of Nuclear Medicine
The Union Memorial Hospital
Baltimore, Maryland

With Illustrations by Lydia V. Kibiuk

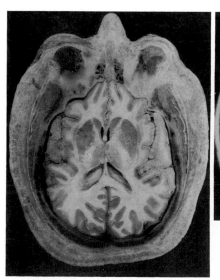

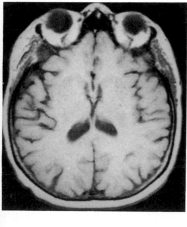

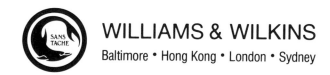

WILLIAMS & WILKINS

Baltimore • Hong Kong • London • Sydney

SANS TACHE

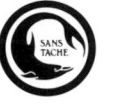

Editor: Laurel Craven
Associate Editor: Victoria M. Vaughn
Copy Editor: Thomas Lehr
Designer: Wilma Rosenberger
Illustration Planner: Wayne Hubbel
Production Coordinator: Barbara J. Felton

Copyright © 1990
Williams & Wilkins
428 East Preston Street
Baltimore, Maryland 21202, USA

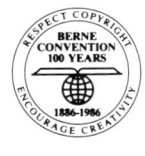

Printed in the United States of America

Library of Congress Cataloging-in-Publication Data

Barrett, Charles P.
    Primer of sectional anatomy with MRI and CT correlation / Charles
P. Barrett, Steven J. Poliakoff, Lawrence E. Holder ; with
illustrations by Lydia V. Kibiuk.
      p.   cm.
    ISBN 0-683-00471-9
    1. Anatomy, Human—Atlases. 2. Magnetic resonance imaging—
Atlases. 3. Tomography—Atlases.   I. Poliakoff, Steven J.
II. Holder, Lawrence E. III. Title.
    [DNLM: 1. Anatomy, Regional—atlases. 2. Magnetic Resonance
Imaging—atlases. 3. Tomography, X-Ray Computed—atlases.   QS 17
B274P]
QM25.B323 1990
611'.0022'2—dc20
DNLM/DLC
for Library of Congress   89-22677
                                           CIP

90 91 92 93 94
1 2 3 4 5 6 7 8 9 10

To our wives,

Elaine,

Chandralekha,

and

Nancy

Acknowledgments

We have had much help in the various stages of the primer project and we are grateful to many people. At The Union Memorial Hospital: a very special thanks is extended to Ken Ballou, B.S., C.N.M.T., Supervisor, Department of Magnetic Resonance Imaging. The imaging correlations in this primer are largely the result of his patient and tireless efforts. Donna Haggerty was also very helpful in this regard, as was Pat Sauer, and we thank them. We also gratefully acknowledge the professional assistance of the radiologists specializing in MR imaging at the Union Memorial Hospital: Dr. Jerry Patt, Director; Drs. Larry Greif, Carlton Sexton, Tom Snider, Andrew Yang, and Ed Steiner. Drs. Sexton and Steiner were particularly helpful with the image correlation. At the University of Maryland, we thank William Parkent of the Anatomy Department, whose invaluable help and suggestions in many of the technical aspects of the preparation of material and photography were indispensable. The cooperation and assistance of Ron Wade, Director of the Anatomy Board of the State of Maryland, and Fred Bland, Administrator of the Department of Anatomy, are appreciated and acknowledged, as are the encouragement and advice given by Drs. Lloyd Guth, Chairman of the Department of Anatomy, and Rosemary Rees, Director of Gross Anatomy. Finally, a word of thanks to all the people at Williams & Wilkins for their more than considerable help and advice.

List of Plates

Section III. Coronal Sections of the Head

Section IV. Transaxial Sections of the Thorax

Section V. Transaxial Sections of the Abdomen

Section VI. Transaxial Sections of the Pelvis

Section VII. Transaxial Sections of the Extremities

Introduction

One of the major goals of courses in gross anatomy is to impart first-hand knowledge of the size, shape, and three-dimensional relationships of the parts of the body. This goal can be optimally achieved by studying sectional anatomy in conjunction with traditional dissection. The purpose of this primer is to introduce basic sectional anatomy using cadaver specimens. It also introduces applied sectional anatomy using magnetic resonance (MR) images and x-ray computerized axial tomographs (CT scans).

The primer is arranged into seven sections, each consisting of a number of plates in which a slice of cadaver material is presented with comparable MR images or CT scans. Major anatomical and clinically relevant structures are identified, with more detail available or deducible by reference to figures found in two standard atlases: *Grant's Atlas of Anatomy, 8th edition* James E. Anderson, ed. (Baltimore, Williams & Wilkins, 1983) and *Color Atlas of Anatomy, 2nd edition* Johannes W. Rohen and Chirhiro Yokochi (New York, Igaku-Shoin). The letter "G" referring to Grant's Atlas is followed by the section and figure number. For example, G 1-7 would indicate Section 1, figure 7. Similarly, the letters "RY" referring to Rohen and Yokochi's Atlas are followed by the page number. The authors strongly recommend the use of these atlases along with the primer and actual cadaver specimens. In this way, the two-dimensional depictions presented by the atlases can be more easily visualized in three dimensions. Further, the nerve and blood vessel relationships omitted in this primer can be appreciated.

Following several sections of the primer, a series of sequential MR images or CT scans is presented as a means for review of the material presented in the section. Viewing and studying the changing patterns of various structures in the individual images or scans in the plate make it possible to mentally synthesize and visualize the overall structure of the region presented in this way. It is also important to note that, in clinical practice, sequential images or slices spaced 0.5–1 cm apart are commonly used to trace the longitudinal course of different structures, as well as to evaluate the extent and location of tumors or other disease processes.

Conventions Used in the Primer

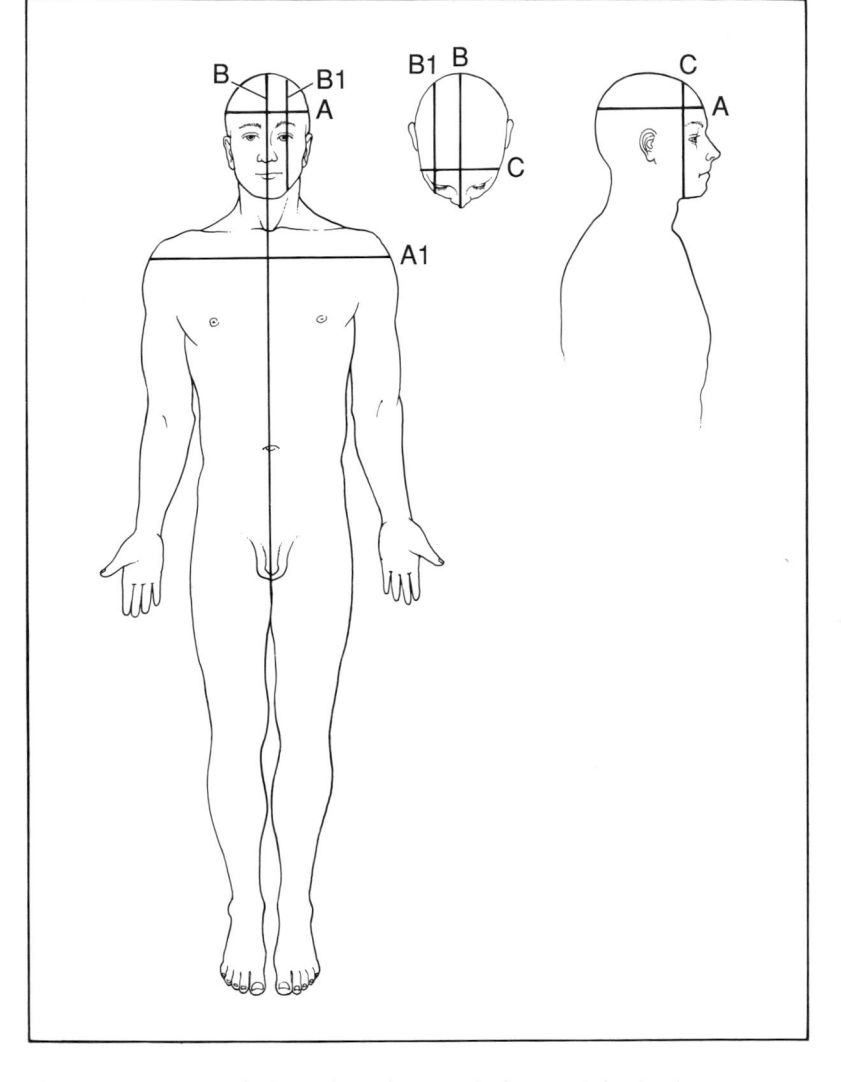

The sections shown in this primer are in the transaxial, sagittal, and coronal planes. The location and plane of each plate are indicated in the diagram accompanying each plate. Each plate is described in terms of three arbitrary points in the section. The various planes are presented in Figure 1. Note that in some cases there is a certain degree of obliqueness relative to the standard planes mentioned; this is also indicated in the diagrams accompanying the plates.

Each plate, except the review plates, contains an anatomical section referred to in the descriptive text as "**A**" and either an MR image or CT scan referred to as "**B**." When feasible, structures visible in both **A** and **B** are labeled. However, no attempt has been made to "force the anatomy" on the electronic images (i.e, the plates labeled **B**). When there is doubt about the anatomy or when the technique does not optimally demonstrate a structure, reference is made to the "region" of the particular structure.

Anatomical and electronic images used in the primer are presented with the cadaver or patient in the standard anatomical position. Transaxial images and sections are oriented as if viewed from below, that is, looking up from the cadaver's or patient's feet; coronal images and sections are viewed from in front of the body, and sagittal images and sections are viewed from the left side of the body.

Figure 1. Transaxial, sagittal, and coronal planes of the body.

Transaxial plane. "Transaxial" is preferred to the terms "cross" or "horizontal" when describing planes of section. It refers to a plane that cuts perpendicular to the axial line of the part being described. Planes *A* and *A1* are examples.

Sagittal plane. This refers to any plane at or parallel to the median plane of the body. Planes *B* and *B1* are examples.

Coronal or frontal plane. This refers to planes that are perpendicular to the median plane of the body (*B* in the figure). Plane *C* is an example.

T1 Weighted		T2 Weighted
Bright High Signal		**Bright High Signal**
1 Fat		CSF, water 1
2 Marrow		2
3		3
4		Intervertebral disk 4
5 Brain, white matter		Brain, gray matter 5
6		6
7 Liver; pancreas		Spleen 7
8 Brain, gray matter		8
9 Kidney		9
10 Spleen		10
11		11
12		Brain, white matter 12
13		Liver 13
14 Cerebrospinal fluid		Fat 14
15 Water; lung		Iron, in basal ganglia 15
16 Bone, cortical; flowing blood, air		Bone, air, flowing blood 16
Dark, low signal		**Dark, low signal**

Figure 2. Comparison of signal intensities in data generated by T1 vs. T2 weighting.

Magnetic resonance (MR) imaging is the correlative imaging modality predominantly used in this book. Conceptually quite different from x-ray imaging techniques, it produces images displayed in standard sagittal, coronal, and transaxial projections.

MR imaging records data based on the magnetic properties of hydrogen nuclei, which can be thought of as tiny magnets spinning in random directions. These nuclei (magnets) interact with neighboring atoms and with externally applied magnetic fields. When an outside source of strong magnetic energy is applied to small magnetic fields they lie parallel to the direction of the external magnet. Radio waves from a secondary coil are then directed at the nuclei from another angle. The nuclei absorb this energy and flip 180° from their previous positions. Cessation of the secondary pulse results in a gradual return of the nuclei to their original, parallel state imposed by the magnet. The energy they release in doing so is measured electronically and analyzed by sophisticated computer algorithms to create a two-dimensional image depicting a thin tissue slice. Depending on their chemical environment, atoms require different amounts of energy to flip and require different times to return to their original orientation. For example, hydrogen in water gives off a different spectrum than hydrogen in protein or fat. Since water and fat content varies from tissue to tissue or between a collection of tumor cells surrounding normal cells, differences in released energy can be used to diagnose the presence of abnormalities within organs also. T1 and T2 relaxation times are two measures of these energy absorbing and releasing characteristics. By altering parameters associated with data generation, images can be produced that emphasize one or the other of these characteristics. In this primer, the images have been created using either T1 or T2 characteristics of the tissues, called T1 or T2 weighting. The *relative* gray scale positions of various tissues in images obtained with T1 or T2 weighting are illustrated in Figure 2.

The other imaging modality used in this primer, computed or computerized tomography (CT scanning), is an x-ray-based technique in which x-ray photons interact with a scintillation crystal that is more sensitive than x-ray film. Sophisticated computers and programs applying algorithms similar to those used for MR imaging generate representative transaxial images. Display of CT images generally reflects the gradation between four basic densities: *air* (black), *fat* (dark/gray), *water/blood* (gray/light), and *bone/metal* (white). Currently, CT scanning is the method of choice for abdominal studies, since patients are usually able to hold their breath for the 2 seconds of data acquisition required for each slice, thus eliminating the image degradation associated with respiratory motion. The longer data acquisition times of MR imaging create technical difficulties in this regard. The choice of which imaging modality to use, in general, is dictated by the nature of the tissue under examination. For example, bone marrow can be better characterized on MR images than on CT scans. However, bone detail is better seen on CT scans.

Preparation
of Anatomical Specimens

The anatomical specimens used in this primer were prepared by freezing embalmed cadavers for approximately 1 week and then sectioning them with a bandsaw. Following sectioning, specimens were further prepared by washing them under a stream of warm water and, in most cases, dissecting blood and other material from blood vessels and hollow organs before photography.

Primer of
Sectional Anatomy with MRI and CT Correlation

PLATE 1. Transaxial section through frontal sinus, splenium of corpus callosum, and superior sagittal sinus, T1 MR image

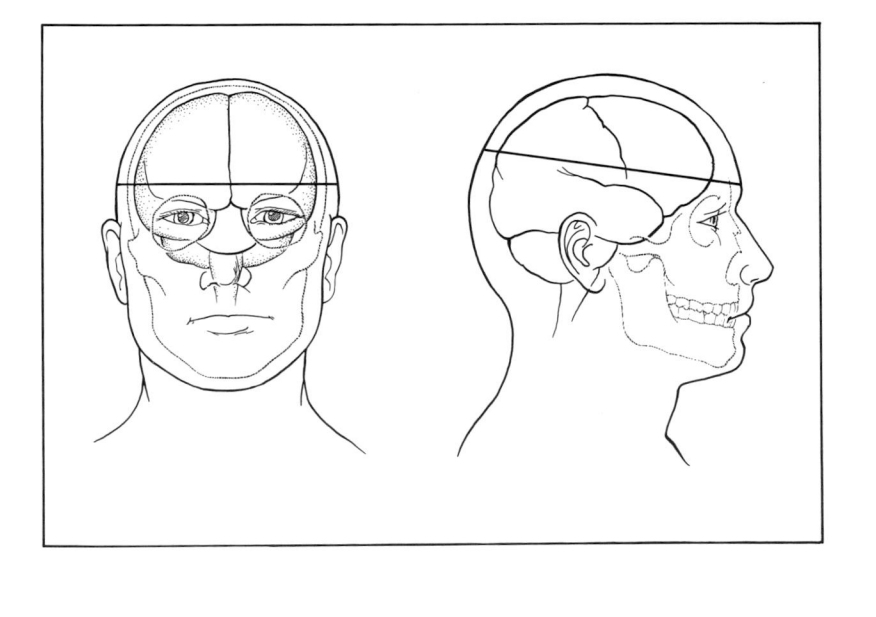

Note

- **Frontal** (*F*), **parietal** (*P*), and **occipital** (*O*) lobes of the cerebrum.
- The mucoperiosteal-lined **frontal sinuses.**
- The **superior sagittal fissure** separating the left and right frontal lobes of the cerebrum anteriorly and the parietal lobes posteriorly.
- The **genu** (*G*), **splenium**, and **trunk (body)** of the **corpus callosum**, the trunk forming the roof of the **lateral ventricles**.
- The **caudate nucleus** (*CN*) protruding as the lateral wall into the cavity of the body of the **lateral ventricle.**
- The **anterior cerebral artery** anterior to the **genu** (*G*) of the **corpus callosum.**
- The **anterior horn** of the **lateral ventricle** and the **periventricular white matter** (*).
- The **superior sagittal sinus** formed by the inner layer and the outer or periosteal layer of dura mater.
- In **B**, the **central sulcus** of the cerebrum outlined by cerebrospinal fluid (CSF).
- In **B**, the bony **inner** and **outer tables** of the **calvaria**, and between them the bright signal of the **diploë** (cancellous bone interspersed with hematopoietic and fatty marrow).

Clinical Notes

- Magnetic resonance (MR) imaging is the most sensitive technique for visualizing intracerebral pathology.
- Clinically, T1 images are used to detect the bright signal of subacute hemorrhage. T2 images of the cerebrum are anatomically striking and often most sensitive for detection of disease.
- Periventricular white matter tract lesions occurring in multiple sclerosis and other demyelinating diseases are well seen in MR images.

References: G 7–19, 7–30A; RY 84, 100–101, 112

Frontal sinus

Superior sagittal fissure

Anterior cerebral artery
Anterior horn of lateral ventricle

Trunk of corpus callosum

Splenium of corpus callosum

Calvaria

Superior sagittal sinus

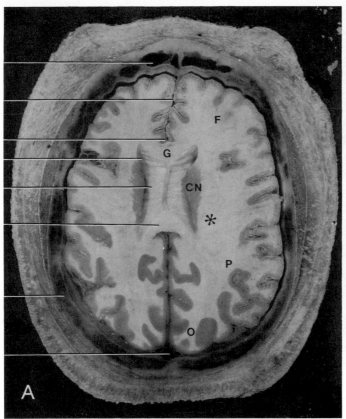

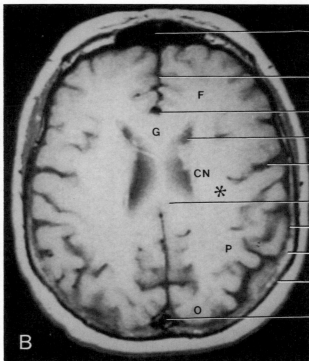

Frontal sinus

Superior sagittal fissure

Anterior cerebral artery

Anterior horn of
 lateral ventricle
Central sulcus

Splenium of corpus callosun

Inner table of calvaria

Diploë

Outer table of calvaria

Superior sagittal sinus

CN-caudate nucleus
F-frontal lobe
G-genu of corpus callosum
O-occipital lobe

P-parietal lobe
asterisk-periventricular white
　　　　matter

PLATE 2. Transaxial section through orbit, internal capsule, and superior sagittal sinus, T1 MR image

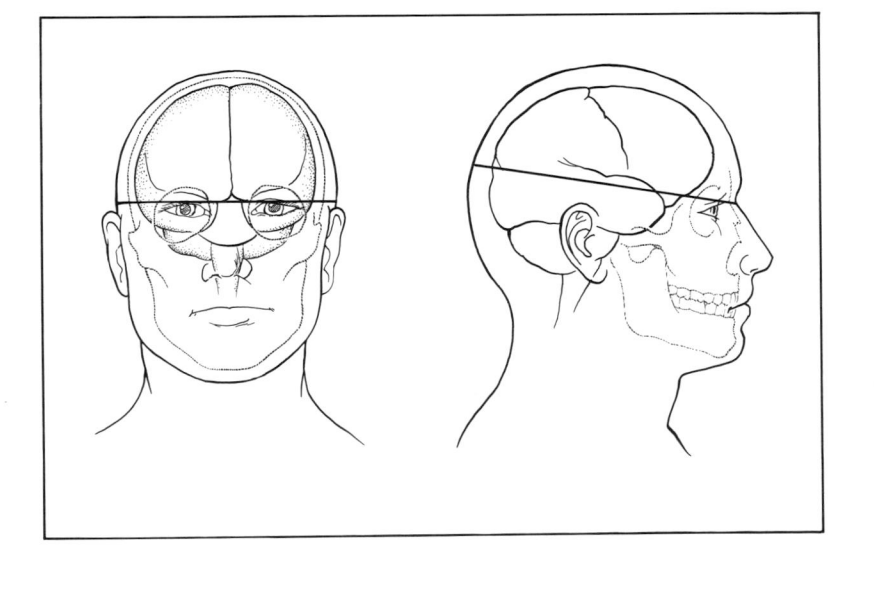

Note

- The **frontal** (*F*) **insular** (**insula**) (*I*), **temporal** (*T*), **parietal** (*P*) and **occipital** (*O*) lobes of the cerebrum.
- The **lateral ventricle** labeled near its posterior horn, posterior to which lies the **splenium** (*S*) of the corpus callosum.
- The thin, lateral wall of the **ethmoid sinus**, forming the medial wall of the orbit.
- The **transverse cerebral fissure** (**sylvian fissure**), outlined by cerebrospinal fluid (CSF) in **B**.
- The cavity of the **third ventricle**, between the left and the right **thalamus** (*TH*).
- The **superior sagittal sinus**.
- In **A**, the interventricular foramina to the left and right of the **fornix columns**.
- In **A**, the V-shaped **internal capsule** (*CP*) and the surrounding **head of caudate nucleus** (*CN*), **putamen** (*PT*), and **thalamus** (*TH*).
- In **B**, the bright signal of **periorbital fat**.
- In **B**, the **anterior cerebral artery** in the superior sagittal fissure.

Clinical Notes

- Hypertensive-induced hemorrhage commonly occurs in the basal ganglia and is manifested as a bright signal on T1 images.
- Although structures around the internal capsule are indistinct in this MR image, it is possible to vary display parameters to clearly separate the basal ganglia and thalamus on T1 images. T2-weighted images, however, will more directly delineate them.

References: G 7–1, 7–30A; RY 84, 100–101, 113

Ethmoid sinus

Temporalis

Transverse cerebral fissure

Fornix columns

Third ventricle

Lateral ventricle

Superior sagittal sinus

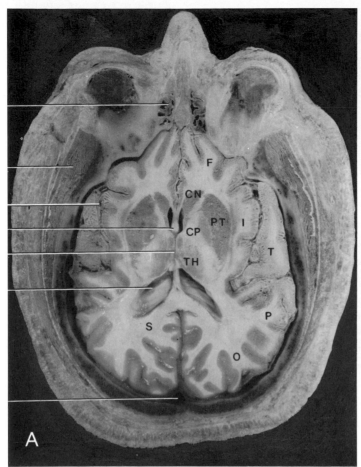

A

Ethmoid sinus

Periorbital fat

Anterior cerebral artery

Transverse cerebral fissure
Third ventricle

Lateral ventricle

Inner table of calvaria

Diploë

Outer table of calvaria

Superior sagittal sinus

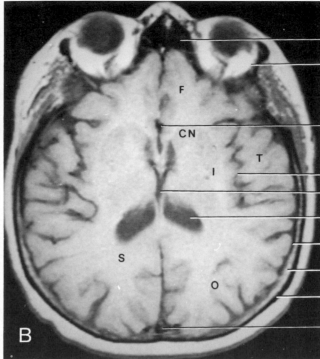

B

CN-caudate nucleus	**F**-frontal lobe	**O**-occipital lobe	**PT**-putamen	**T**-temporal lobe
CP-internal capsule	**I**-insular lobe	**P**-parietal lobe	**S**-splenium of corpus callosum	**TH**-thalamus

PLATE 3. Transaxial section through orbit at the optic nerve, diencephalic-mesencephalic junction, and superior sagittal sinus, T2 MR image

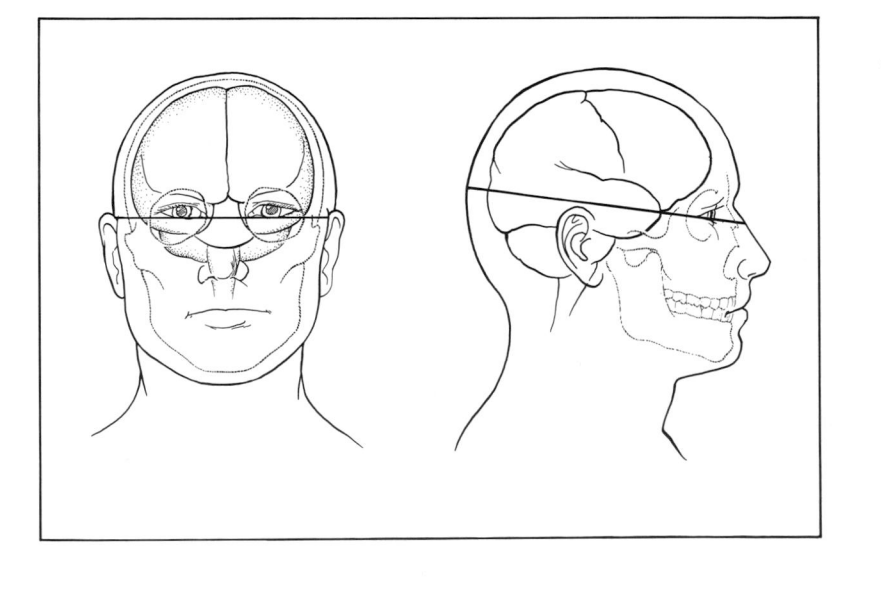

Note

- That the MR image, **B**, is slightly inferior to **A**.
- The **temporal** (*T*), **parietal** (*P*), and **occipital** (*O*) lobes of the cerebrum.
- The **falx cerebri**, separating the **occipital lobes**.
- The **ethmoid sinuses** between the orbits.
- The **optic nerves** converging at right angles to one another.
- The **lateral rectus muscle**, in **B** giving a dark signal and thus being clearly differentiated from the bright signal of periorbital fat.
- The **lateral ventricle** labeled near its posterior horn, and its contents, the cerebrospinal fluid (CSF), giving a bright signal in this T2 MR image
- In **B**, the **middle cerebral artery** in its lateral course between the **temporal** and **frontal** lobes of the cerebrum.

Clinical Notes

- The appearance of the middle cerebral artery in **B** shows that blood vessels may be distinguished by MR imaging without using intravenous contrast injections.
- Obstruction of the internal carotid artery can be diagnosed by MR imaging because of the difference in signal between clotted (*light gray*) and free-flowing blood (*black*).

References: G 7–1; RY 84, 115

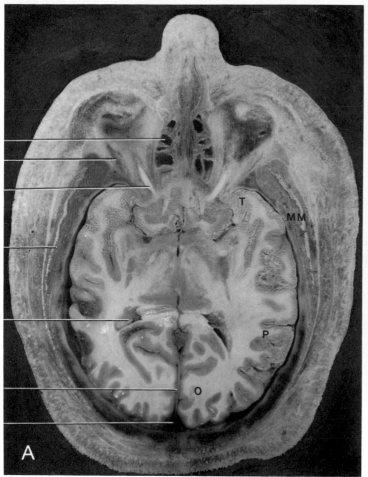

Ethmoid sinus

Lateral rectus

Optic nerve

Temporalis

Lateral ventricle

Falx cerebri

Superior sagittal sinus

A

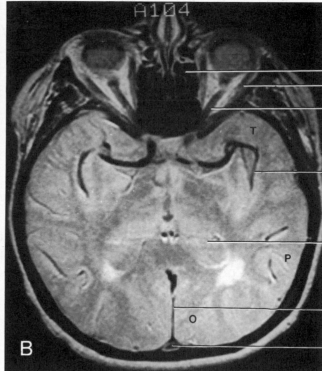

Ethmoid sinus

Lateral rectus

Optic nerve

Middle cerebral artery

Lateral ventricle

Falx cerebri

Superior sagittal sinus

B

O-occipital lobe
P-parietal lobe
T-temporal lobe

Section I. PLATE 3. *Orbit at the Optic Nerve, Diencephalic-Mesencephalic Junction, Superior Sagittal Sinus* 7

PLATE 4. Transaxial section through the middle nasal concha, sphenoid sinus, and superior sagittal sinus, T2 MR image

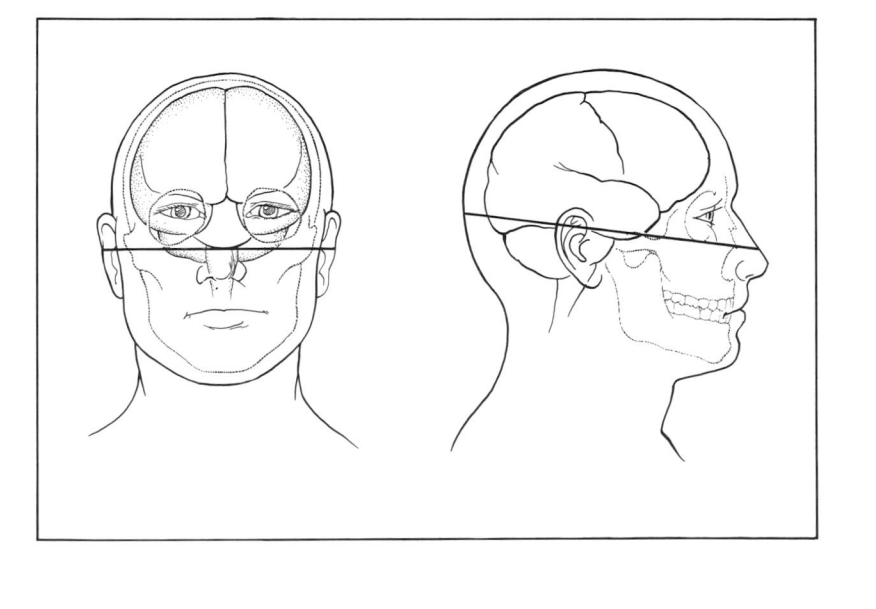

Note

- That **A** is slightly inferior to **B.**
- The **temporal** (*T*) and **occipital** (*O*) lobes of the cerebrum.
- The **vermis of the cerebellum** (*VC*).
- The **cerebral aqueduct**, passing through the **mesencephalon.**
- In **A**, the roof of the **maxillary sinus** appearing just inferior to and thus forming part of the floor of the orbit, compared to **B,** which lies just superior to the floor of the orbit.
- The highly vascular, mucoperiosteal-lined **middle nasal concha.**
- The **sphenoid sinus,** whose roof (see in **A**) lies just inferior to the hypophyseal fossa.
- The **basilar artery,** posterior to the **clivus** (*white dashes*) and anterior to the cerebral penduncles of the **mesencephalon** (*M*) in **A** and to the **pons** (*PO*) in **B.**
- The **falx cerebri** and the **superior sagittal sinus**.

Clinical Notes

- The middle meningeal artery (*MM*) is vulnerable to laceration in fractures of the temporal bone. Hemorrhage from the torn vessel may lead to epidural hematoma, which is detectable in MR images.
- Because of its sensitivity, MR imaging is the modality of choice in evaluating temporal lobe lesions.
- MR imaging is also optimal for evaluation of the cerebrum, cerebellum, and brainstem in the posterior cranial fossa since it eliminates bone artifacts present with CT scans. It is useful in revealing brainstem infarctions, neoplasms, and demyelinating diseases such as multiple sclerosis.

References: G 7–49, 7–105; RY 84, 114, section 4, 132

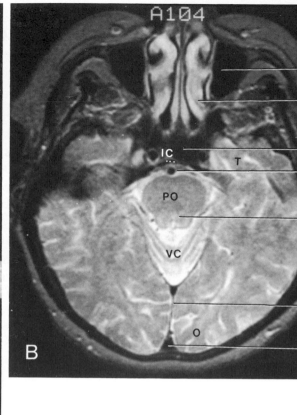

Facial vein

Maxillary sinus

Middle nasal concha

Sphenoid sinus

Basilar artery

Temporalis

Cerebral aqueduct

Falx cerebri

Superior sagittal sinus

A

Maxillary sinus

Middle nasal concha

Sphenoid sinus

Basilar artery

Cerebral aqueduct

Falx cerebri

Superior sagittal sinus

B

A104

IC · · · CPE · T · MM · M · VC · O

PO · VC · IC · T · O

IC-internal carotid artery **MM**-middle meningeal artery **PO**-pons **VC**-cerebellar vermis
CPE-cerebral peduncles **O**-occipital lobe **T**-temporal lobe **White dots**-clivus
M-mesencephalon

Section I. PLATE 4. *Middle Nasal Concha, Sphenoid Sinus, and Superior Sagittal Sinus* 9

PLATE 5. Transaxial section through the inferior nasal concha, pons, and cerebellum, T2 MR image

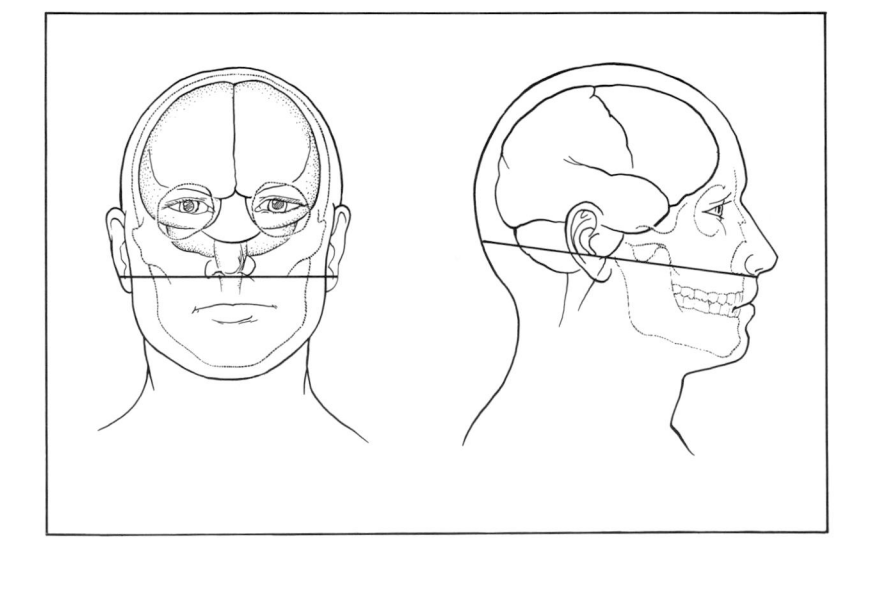

Note

- The **occipital lobe** (O) of the **cerebrum** (**A** only) and the **vermis** (VC) and **lateral lobes** (LC) of the **cerebellum**.
- The **maxillary sinus** lateral to the **inferior nasal concha**, posterior to which lies the **nasopharynx** (NP).
- The **head of the mandible** and the **lateral pterygoid muscle** coursing toward it.
- The **internal carotid artery** (IC) in the carotid canal.
- In **A**, the cavity of the **fourth ventricle** (IV) between the **vermis** of the cerebellum and the **pons** (PO).
- In **A**, the continuity between the **external acoustic meatus**, the **middle ear** (ME), and the **auditory tube** (AT) leading to the **nasopharynx** (NP), and the proximity of the **mastoid air cells** to the **middle ear**.
- In **A**, the **basilar artery** (BA) lying posterior to the **clivus** (CL) and anterior to the **pons** (PO).
- In **A**, the **straight sinus** between the **lateral lobes of the cerebellum**.
- In **A**, the underside of the **tentorium cerebelli** separating the **cerebellum** from the **occipital lobe** of the **cerebrum**.
- In **A**, the **transverse sinus** at its termination in the sigmoid sinus.

Clinical Notes

- In **A**, the relationships that explain the spread of infection from the nasopharynx into the auditory tube, middle ear, and mastoid air cells can be seen.
- The soft tissue planes of the nasopharynx as seen in this MR image are used in the evaluation of nasopharyngeal masses.
- Special MR image views of the temporomandibular joint are used to identify joint disk pathology.

References: G 7–1; RY 84, 114

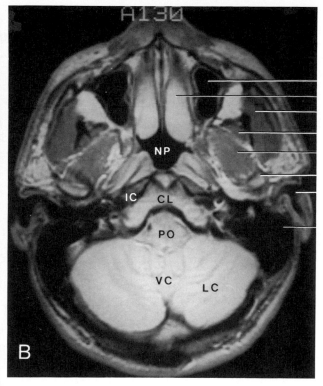

Maxillary sinus

Masseter

Temporalis

Lateral pterygoid

Head of mandible

External acoustic meatus

Mastoid air cells

Transverse sinus

Tentorium cerebelli
Straight sinus

Superior sagittal sinus

A

NP

AT

CL

ME

BA

IC

PO

+IV

VC

LC

O

Maxillary sinus
Inferior nasal concha
Masseter

Temporalis

Lateral pterygoid

Head of mandible
External acoustic meatus

Mastoid air cells

B

NP

IC

CL

PO

VC

LC

AT-auditory tube   IC-internal carotid artery   LC-lateral lobe of cerebellum   NP-nasopharynx   PO-pons
BA-basilar artery   IV-fourth ventricle   ME-middle ear   O-occipital lobe   VC-vermis of cerebellum
CL-clivus

PLATE 6. Transaxial section through hard palate, nasopharynx, and internal occipital protuberance, T2 MR image

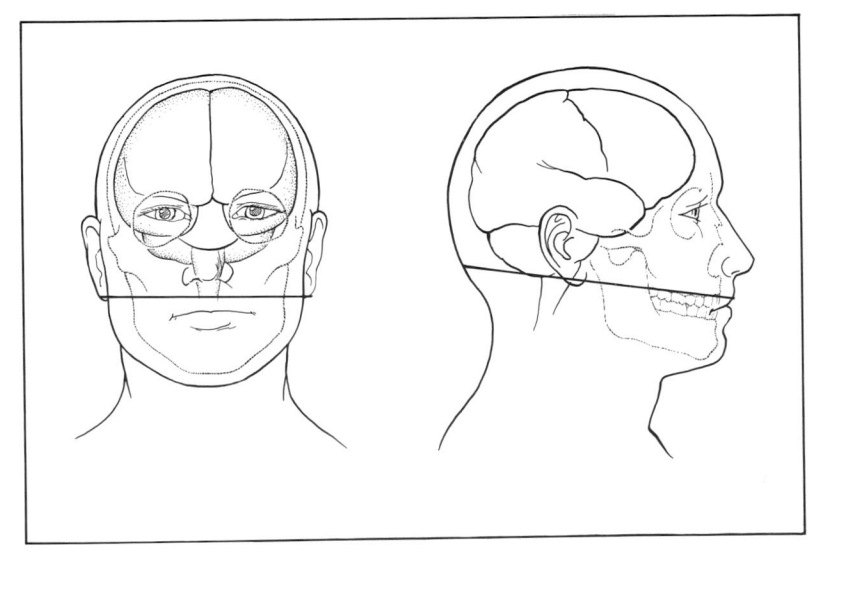

Note

- That **B** is slightly inferior to **A**.
- The **lateral lobes** (*LC*) of the cerebellum.
- The infratemporal region medial to the ramus of the **mandible** with the **medial pterygoid muscle** and branches of the **maxillary artery** (*MA*).
- The **parotid gland** (*PG*) posterior and medial to the ramus of the **mandible** overlapping the **masseter muscle** laterally.
- The **internal carotid artery** (in **A**, *IC*) and **internal jugular vein,** the latter in **A** having just received the termination of the **sigmoid sinus** (*SI*).
- The **vertebral arteries** (*VA*) posterior to the **clivus** and anterior to the **medulla oblongata** (*MO*) at the level of the **fourth ventricle** in **A** and the **cerebellomedullary cistern** (**cisterna magna**) in **B**.
- The **mastoid air cells**, medial to which lies the **jugular foramen**.

Clinical Notes

- Tumors of the parotid and other salivary glands may involve the infratemporal fossa and subsequently invade the parapharyngeal space medial to the pterygoid muscles.

References: G 7–92; RY 155

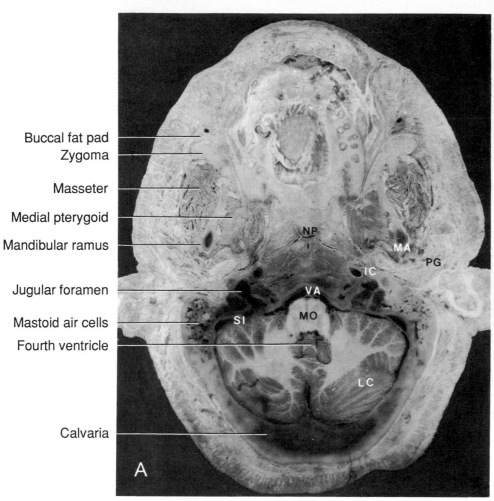

Buccal fat pad

Zygoma

Masseter

Medial pterygoid

Mandibular ramus

Jugular foramen

Mastoid air cells

Fourth ventricle

Calvaria

A

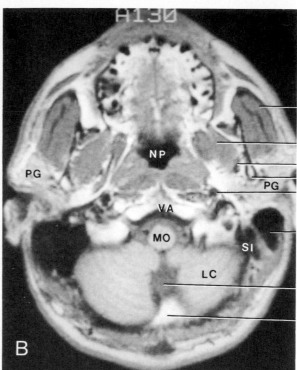

Masseter

Medial pterygoid

Branch of maxillary artery

Mandibular ramus

Internal carotid artery

Mastoid air cells

Cerebellomedullary cistern

Diploic fat

B

IC-internal carotid artery   **MA**-maxillary artery   **NP**-nasopharynx   **SI**-sigmoid sinus
LC-lateral lobe of cerebellum   **MO**-medulla oblongata   **PG**-parotid gland   **VA**-vertebral artery

PLATE 7. Transaxial section through symphysis and body of mandible, oropharynx, and cervical spinal cord, T2 MR image

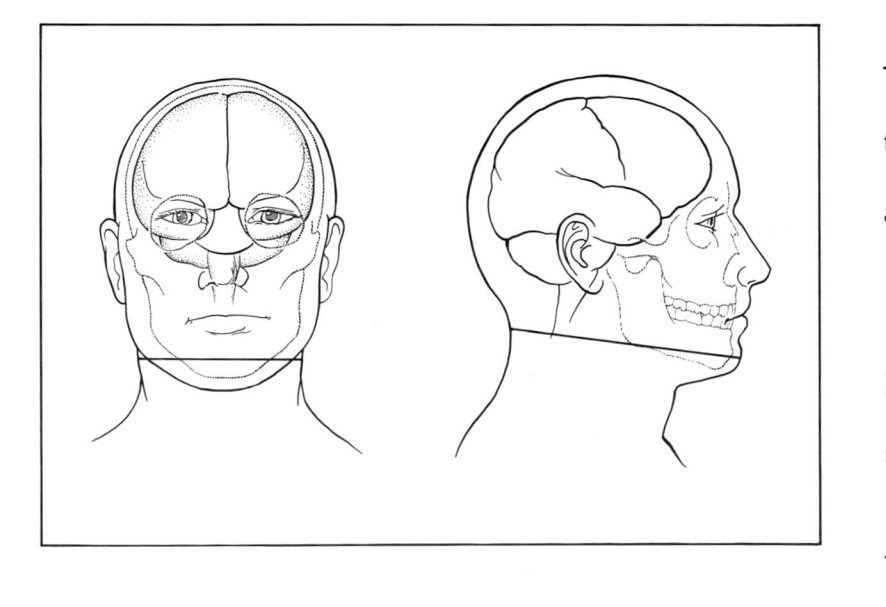

Note

- The **symphysis of the mandible**, and passing posteriorly from it the muscle fibers of the **genioglossus**.
- The **mylohyoid muscle** and its close relationship to the **submandibular gland** (*SM*) and the **sublingual gland** (*SL*).
- The initial segment of the **oropharynx**.
- The **cervical spinal cord** and the surrounding dura mater.
- The **vertebral artery** (*VA*) in the foramen transversarium.
- In **A**, the **internal carotid artery** and lateral to it the **internal jugular vein** (*IJ*); similarly, in **B**, the **internal jugular vein** (*IJ*) lateral to the **common carotid artery** (*CC*).
- Posteriorly and superficially, the **trapezius**, and deep to it the **semispinalis capitis**, **multifidus**, and **splenius capitis** muscles.

Clinical Notes

- The jugulodigastric region (*small circles*) contains many lymph nodes, which are often affected by metastatic head and neck carcinoma. Significant lymphadenopathy may be impalpable, but identification is quite possible with MR imaging or CT scanning.
- MR imaging is useful in detecting lesions within the submandibular gland, tongue, and floor of the mouth and in demonstrating their relationship to the mandible.

References: G 7–1; RY 84, 210

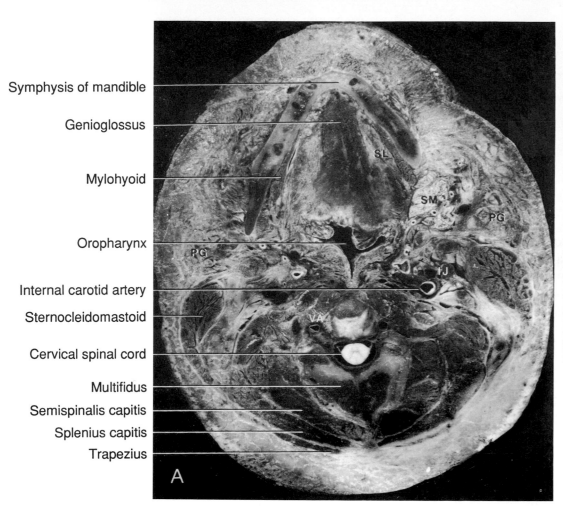

Symphysis of mandible

Genioglossus

Mylohyoid

Oropharynx

Internal carotid artery

Sternocleidomastoid

Cervical spinal cord

Multifidus

Semispinalis capitis

Splenius capitis

Trapezius

A

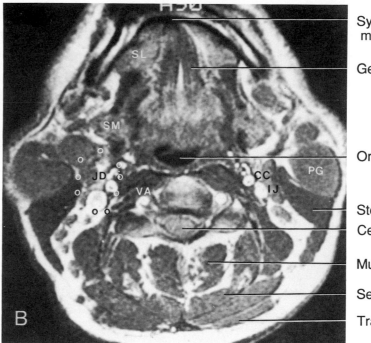

Symphysis of mandible

Genioglossus

Oropharynx

Sternocleidomastoid
Cervical spinal cord

Multifidus

Semispinalis capitis

Trapezius

B

CC-common carotid artery
IJ-internal jugular vein
JD-jugulodigastric region (out-
lined by small white circles)

PG-parotid gland
SL-sublingual gland

SM-submandibular gland
VA-vertebral artery

PLATE 8. Transaxial section through floor of mouth, epiglottis, and cervical spinal cord, T2 MR image

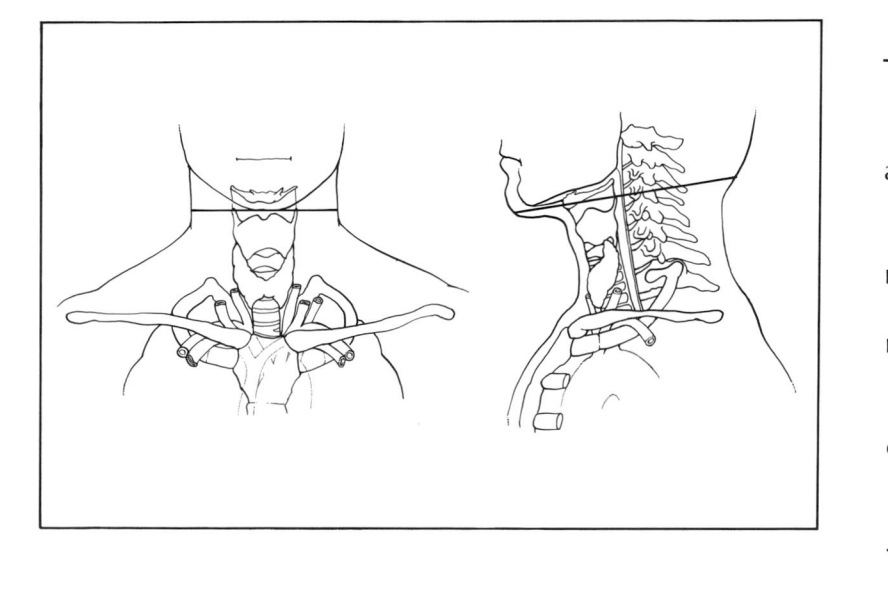

Note

- That **A** is slightly superior to **B**.
- The relative positions of the **common carotid artery** (*CC*), **internal jugular vein** (*IJ*), and **vagus nerve**.
- The **vertebral artery** in the foramen transversarium.
- In **A**, the relative positions of the following muscles: **anterior belly of the digastric**, **mylohyoid**, and **geniohyoid**.
- In **A**, the **submandibular gland** (*SM*) and its close relationship to the **mylohyoid muscle**.
- In **A**, the **lesser** and **greater cornua** of the **hyoid bone**.
- In **A**, the **epiglottis** anterior to the cavity of the **oropharynx**, and in **B**, the **thyroid cartilage** anterior to the cavity of the **larynx**.

Clinical Notes

- The extent of laryngeal carcinoma, readily determinable by MR imaging, is critical in choosing between supraglottic laryngectomy, hemilaryngectomy, and total laryngectomy.

References: G 7–1, 9–34, 9–38, 9–82; RY 84, 142, 143, 160

Anterior belly of digastric

Mylohyoid

Geniohyoid

Lesser cornu of hyoid bone

Epiglottis

Greater cornu of hyoid bone

Middle pharyngeal constrictor

Vagus nerve

Vertebral artery

Multifidus

Semispinalis capitis

Splenius capitis

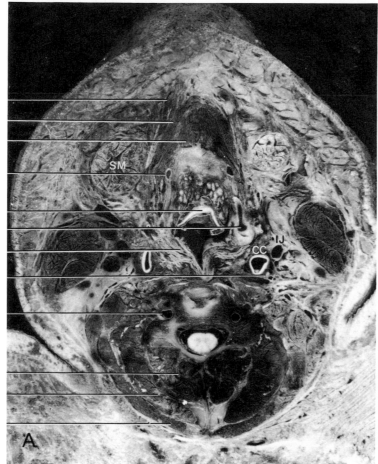

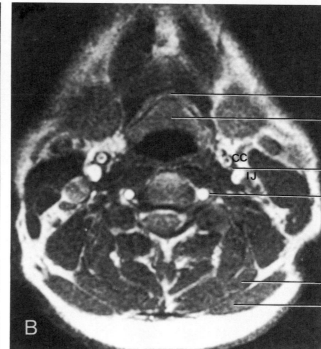

Hyoid bone

Epiglottis

Vagus nerve

Vertebral artery

Semispinalis capitis

Trapezius

CC-common carotid artery
IJ-internal jugular vein
SM-submandibular gland

PLATE 9. Transaxial section through the thyroid cartilage, body of the fifth cervical vertebra, and cervical spinal cord, T2 MR image

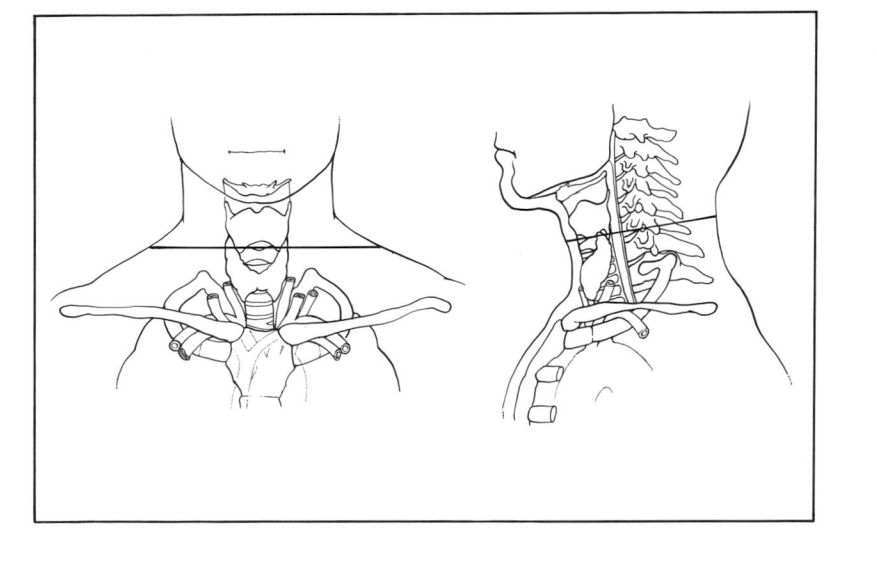

Note

- The lamina of the **thyroid cartilage** and posterior to it the **cavity of the larynx**.
- The posterior wall of the larynx formed by the **cricoid cartilage**.
- The **thyroid gland** and, between it and the **cricoid cartilage, the inferior cornu** of the **thyroid cartilage**.
- The **common carotid artery** (*CC*) and lateral to it the **internal jugular vein** (*IJ*), and between these the **vagus nerve**.
- The **scalenus anterior**, **scalenus medius**, and **longus colli** muscles.
- The **retropharyngeal space** between the buccopharyngeal fascia of the **laryngopharynx** and the prevertebral fascia of the fifth cervical **vertebral body**.
- The **vertebral artery** in the foramen transversarium.

Clinical Notes

- The carotid artery and jugular vein can be traced throughout their slightly oblique course in the neck by using sequential sections. MR imaging has the potential to noninvasively evaluate atheromatous plaque within the carotid artery.
- Degenerative arthritis with bone production can cause narrowing of the spinal canal with resultant cord compression or nerve impingement; such lesions are discernible by use of MR imaging or CT scanning.

References: G 9–3B and C, 9–82 (see also 9–38 presenting a frontal view of the root of the neck); RY 171, 160

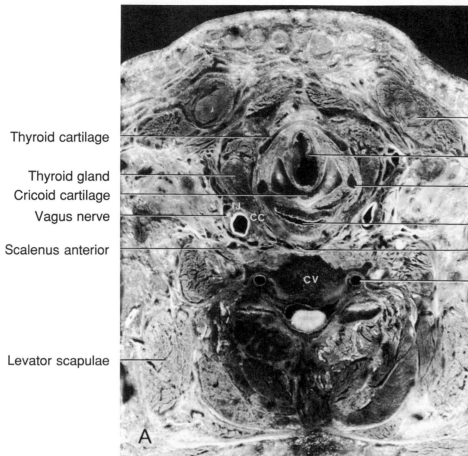

Thyroid cartilage

Thyroid gland
Cricoid cartilage
Vagus nerve

Scalenus anterior

Levator scapulae

Sternocleidomastoid

Vocal folds
Inferior cornu of thyroid cartilage

Laryngopharynx
Retropharyngeal space

Vertebral artery

A

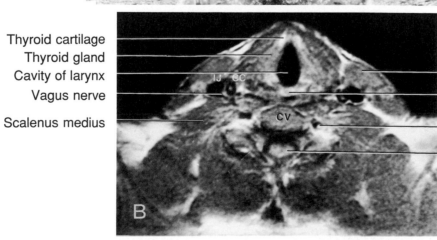

Thyroid cartilage
Thyroid gland
Cavity of larynx
Vagus nerve

Scalenus medius

Sternocleidomastoid

Cricoid cartilage

Vertebral artery

Spinal cord

B

CV-body of fifth cervical vertebra   **CC**-common carotid artery   **IJ**-internal jugular vein

Section I. PLATE 9. *Thyroid Cartilage, Body of Fifth Cervical Vertebra, and Cervical Spinal Cord*   19

PLATE 10. Sagittal section near the midline through the symphysis of the mandible, epiglottis, and fourth ventricle, T1 MR image

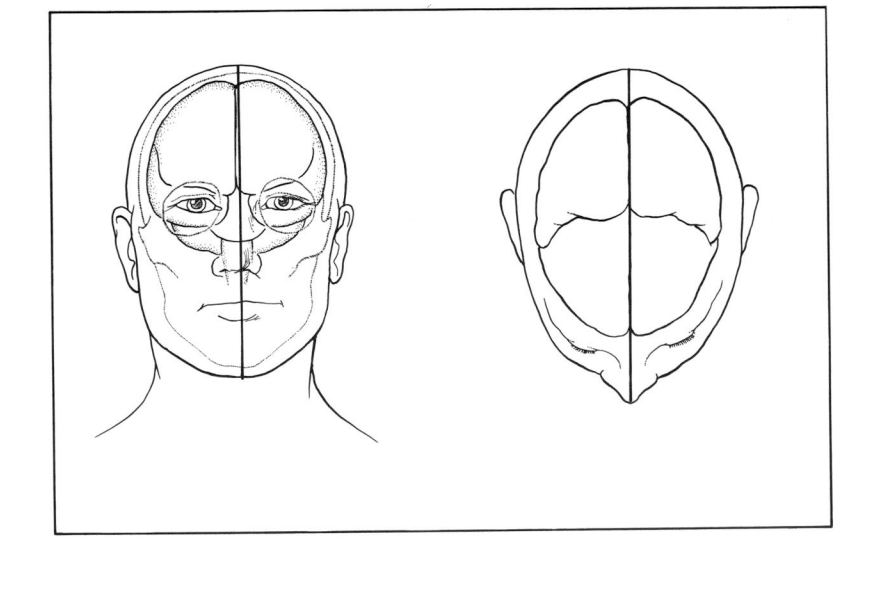

Note

- The **cerebellomedullary cistern** (**cisterna magna**) in the region of the **tonsil, medulla**, and **cervical spinal cord**, outlined by cerebrospinal fluid (CSF) in **B**.
- The **intervertebral disks** between the bodies of the cervical vertebrae.
- Inferior to the **hyoid bone**, the **thyroid cartilage**.
- In **A**, the **odontoid process** (*OP*) and the **anterior** and **posterior arches of the atlas** separated from the spinal canal and **spinal cord** by the **dura mater**, which continues superiorly with the cranial dura mater.
- Posterior to the musculature of the **pharynx** and anterior to the cervical spinal column, the **retropharyngeal space**.
- In **A**, the **epiglottis** at the root of the tongue and posterior to it the musculature of the pharynx.
- In **A**, the **genioglossus muscle** coursing posteriorly from the genial tubercle of the **mandible** to insert into the fascia of the tongue and inferior to it the **geniohyoid** passing to the **hyoid bone**.
- In **A**, central nervous system structures **pons** (*PO*), **medulla oblongata** (*MO*), **cervical spinal cord** (*SC*), **vermis** (*VC*), and **tonsil** (*TO*) of the cerebellum.
- In **B**, the **cavities** of the **trachea** and of the **esophagus**.

Clinical Notes

- The intervertebral disks are well demonstrated in MR images. Degeneration can be diagnosed, and disk protrusion with cord or nerve root impingement can be identified.

References: G 7–1; RY 84; see also Plate 15

Clivus

Vomer

Hard palate

Soft palate

Anterior arch of atlas

Genioglossus

Geniohyoid

Mylohyoid

Epiglottis

Body of hyoid bone

Retropharyngeal space

Laryngopharynx

Thyroid cartilage

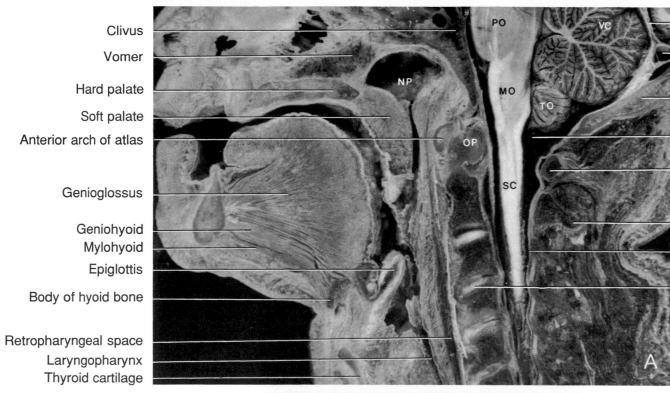

PO

VC

MO

NP

TO

OP

SC

Tentorium cerebelli

Transverse sinus

Occipital bone

Cerebellomedullary cistern

Posterior arch of atlas

Spinous process of axis

Dura mater

Intervertebral disk

A

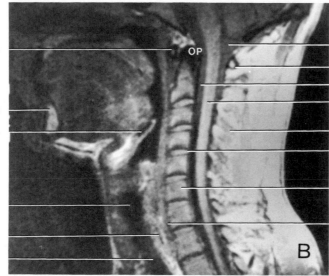

Anterior arch of atlas

Symphysis of mandible

Epiglottis

Larynx

Esophagus

Trachea

OP

Cerebellomedullary cistern

Posterior arch of atlas
Spinal canal
Cervical spinal cord

Cervical spinous process
Intervertebral disk

Body of sixth cervical vertebra

Retropharyngeal space

B

MO-medulla oblongata **PO**-pons **TO**-tonsil of cerebellum
NP-nasopharynx **SC**-cervical spinal cord **VC**-vermis of cerebellum
OP-odontoid process

PLATE 11. Sagittal section through the lateral cerebrum, parotid gland, and mastoid process, T1 MR image

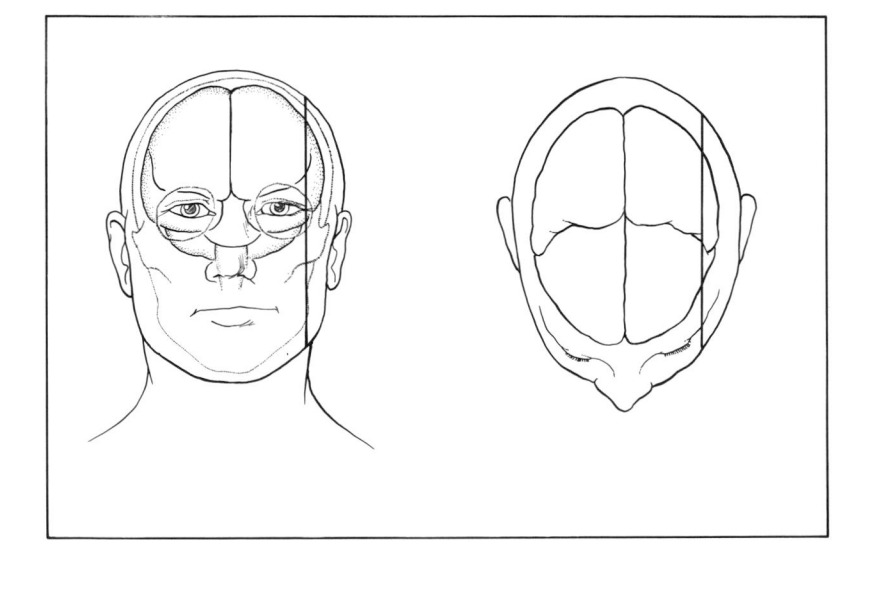

Note

- The **frontal** (*F*), **parietal** (*P*), **temporal** (*T*), and (in **B**) **occipital** (*O*) lobes of the cerebrum.
- The slightly more medial position of **B** relative to **A**, revealing a greater portion of the **masseter muscle**, the **lateral lobe of the cerebellum** (*LC*), and the **occipital lobe** (*O*) of the cerebrum.
- The **parotid gland** inferior and anterior to the **external acoustic meatus** and **mastoid air cells**.
- The **transverse cerebral fissure** (**sylvian fissure**) outlined by cerebrospinal fluid (CSF) in **B**.
- In **A**, part of the **temporalis muscle** superior to the **zygomatic arch** and, inferior to it, part of the **masseter**.

Clinical Notes

- The normal or abnormal parotid gland is well seen by MR imaging.
- Trauma or disease of the parotid gland may compress or destroy branches of the facial nerve within it, resulting in paralysis of facial muscles.

References: G 7–67, 7–71; RY 74–77

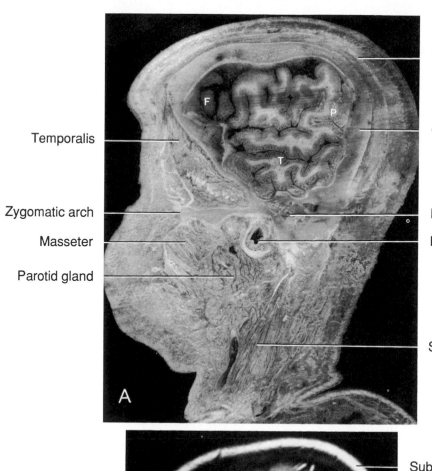

Scalp

Temporalis

Calvaria

Zygomatic arch

Mastoid air cells

Masseter

External acoustic meatus

Parotid gland

Sternocleidomastoid

A

Subcutaneous fat

Central sulcus

Transverse cerebral fissure

Calvaria

Mastoid air cells

Masseter

B

F-frontal lobe   **LC**-lateral lobe of cerebellum   **O**-occipital lobe   **P**-parietal lobe   **T**-temporal lobe

Section II. PLATE 11. *Lateral Cerebrum, Parotid Gland, and Mastoid Process*   23

PLATE 12. Sagittal section through orbit, sigmoid sinus, and transverse process of atlas, T1 MR image

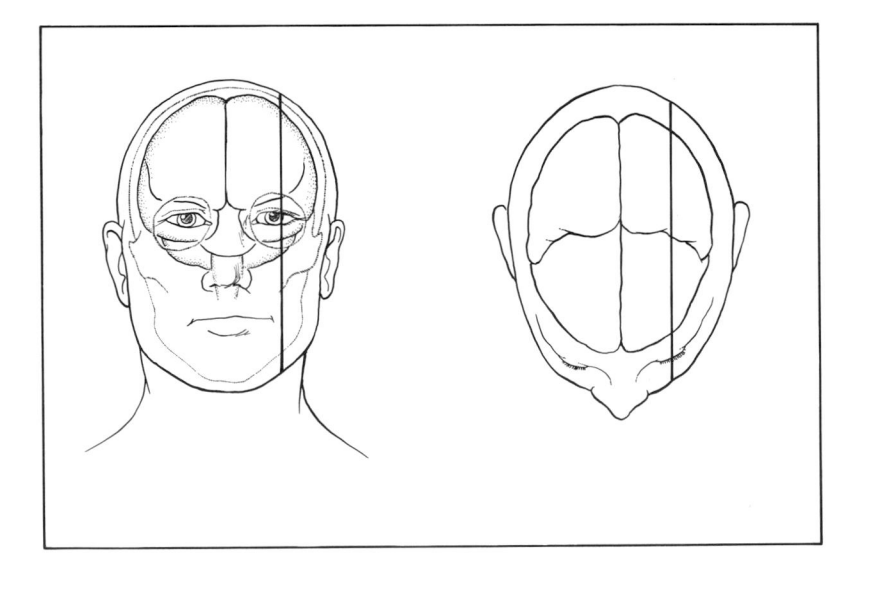

Note

- The **frontal** (*F*), **parietal** (*P*), **occipital** (*O*), **insular** (*I*), and **temporal** (*T*) lobes of the cerebrum.
- The **lateral lobe** (*LC*) of the cerebellum.
- The **maxillary sinus** inferior to the orbit, its posterior wall forming the anterior wall of the infratemporal region containing the **lateral pterygoid muscle** coursing toward the **neck of the mandible** (*NM*).
- In **A**, the five layers of the scalp: **skin, subcutaneous tissue, aponeurosis, loose areolar tissue**, and **pericranium** or **periosteum**.
- In **A**, the **sigmoid sinus** ending at the jugular foramen with the formation of the **internal jugular vein**.
- The **periorbital fat** responsible for the bright signal seen in **B**.
- In **B**, the **petrous temporal bone** and the **mastoid air cells** anterior to the cerebellum.

Clinical Notes

- The location of a lesion as either suprasylvian (frontal or parietal lobes) or infrasylvian (temporal lobe) determines the appropriate neurosurgical approach. The sylvian fissure is well demarcated by sagittal MR imaging. Previously this required angiography, an invasive technique.
- Intraorbital lesions can be located with respect to the low-intensity signal from the globe (*black*) and the high-intensity signal from the periorbital fat (*white*).

References: G 7–21 (layers of scalp), 7–80; RY 70, 79

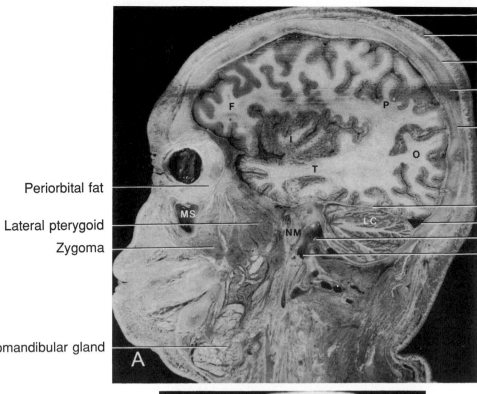

Skin
Subcutaneous tissue
Epicranial aponeurosis
Loose areolar tissue

Pericranium

Periorbital fat

Lateral pterygoid

Zygoma

Tentorium cerebelli
Transverse sinus
Sigmoid sinus
Internal jugular vein

Submandibular gland

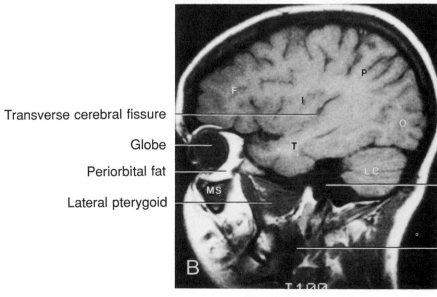

Transverse cerebral fissure

Globe

Periorbital fat

Lateral pterygoid

Petrous temporal bone/mastoid air cells

Angle of mandible

F-frontal lobe
I-insular lobe

LC-lateral lobe of cerebellum
MS-maxillary sinus

NM-neck of mandible
O-occipital lobe

P-parietal lobe
T-temporal lobe

PLATE 13. Sagittal section through orbit, medial part of temporal lobe, and confluence of sinuses, T1 MR image

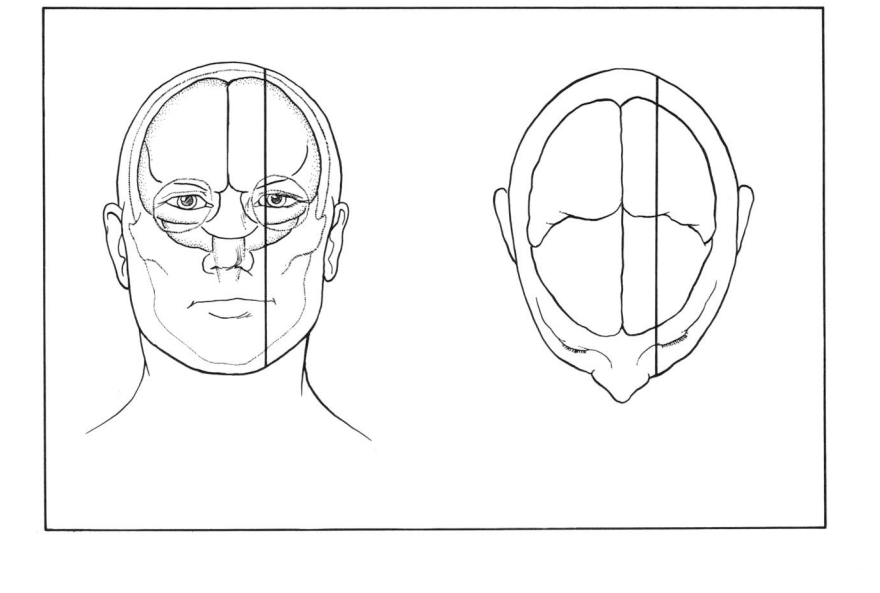

Note

- The **frontal** (*F*), **parietal** (*P*), **occipital** (*O*), and **temporal** (*T*) lobes of the cerebrum, whose sulci in **B** are outlined by cerebrospinal fluid (CSF).
- The **caudate nucleus** (*CN*), **internal capsule** (*CP*), and **pulvinar** (*PU*).
- The **lateral ventricle** sectioned near its posterior horn where it extends as the **temporal horn** into the **temporal lobe**.
- The **frontal sinus** superior to the orbit and the **maxillary sinus** inferior to the orbit.
- The thin **orbital plate** (in **B**, *OP*) of the frontal bone forming the roof of the orbit.
- The **internal carotid artery** in the carotid canal.
- In **A**, the **vertebral artery** sectioned along its course superior to the transverse process of the atlas.
- In **A**, the **tentorium cerebelli** separating the cerebellum from the cerebrum.
- In **B**, the **periorbital fat** appearing as a bright signal, with the darker signal of the **inferior rectus muscle** in marked contrast to it.
- In **B**, the **calvaria** with the **diploë** or cancellous medullary bone containing hematopoietic and fatty marrow.
- In **B**, surrounding the **calvaria**, the bright signal caused by **subcutaneous fat**.

Clinical Notes

- Lesions of the crown of the head (vertex) may arise in subcutaneous tissues, in the diploë, or in the intracranial compartment. Intracranial lesions are intraaxial if they are in cerebral substance and extraaxial if they are in the meninges or in the cerebrospinal fluid–containing spaces (subarachnoid space or any of its cisternal expansions).
- Orbital tumors or masses visible in MR images may arise intraconally (hemangioma, optic nerve meningioma), conally (thyroid ophthalmopathy with muscle enlargement), and extraconally (sinus or lacrimal gland neoplasms).

References: G 7–55 (maxillary sinus and orbital region); RY 106 (lateral ventricle region)

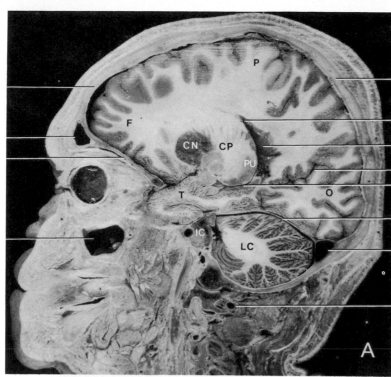

Calvaria

Frontal sinus
Orbital plate of frontal bone

Maxillary sinus

Diploë

Body of lateral ventricle

Posterior horn of lateral ventricle

Calcarine fissure
Temporal horn of lateral ventricle

Tentorium cerebelli

Confluence of sinuses

Vertebral artery

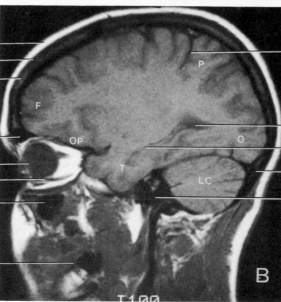

Subcutaneous fat
Outer table of calvaria
Diploë

Frontal sinus

Globe
Inferior rectus

Maxillary sinus

Molar tooth

Central sulcus

Posterior horn of lateral ventricle
Temporal horn of lateral ventricle

Confluence of sinuses

Petrous temporal bone

CN-caudate nucleus   **F**-frontal lobe   **LC**-lateral lobe of cerebellum   **OP**-orbital plate of frontal bone   **PU**-pulvinar
CP-internal capsule   **IC**-internal carotid artery   **O**-occipital lobe   **P**-parietal lobe   **T**-temporal lobe

PLATE 14. Sagittal section through the middle nasal concha, apex of the orbit, and calcarine fissure of the occipital lobe, T1 MR image

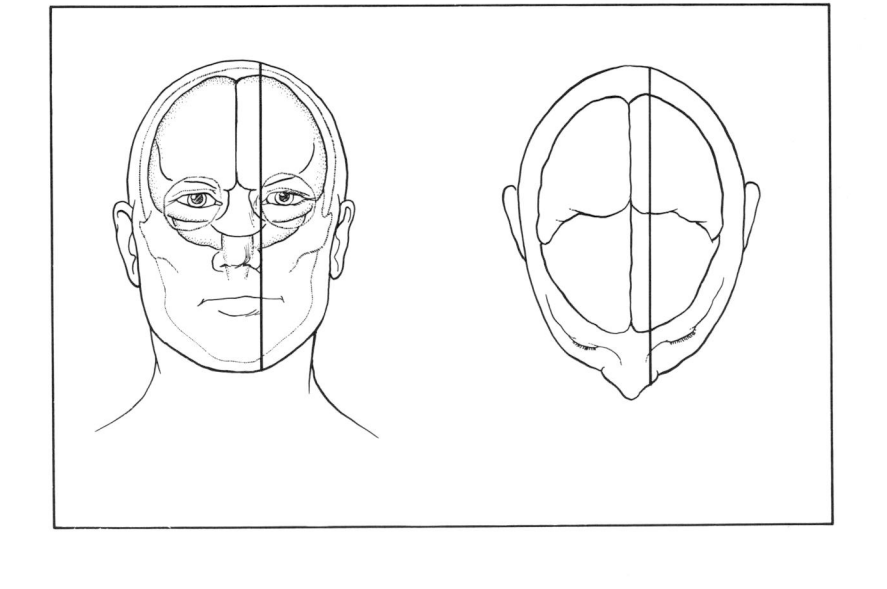

Note

- That **A** is slightly medial to **B**.
- The **frontal** (*F*), **parietal** (*P*), **occipital** (*O*), and **temporal** (*T*) lobes of the cerebrum.
- The **frontal sinus** superior to the orbit.
- The **lateral ventricle** near its posterior horn extending as the **temporal horn** into the temporal lobe.
- In **A**, the **caudate nucleus** (*CN*), **internal capsule** (*CP*), and **pulvinar** (*PU*) lying anterior to the **lateral ventricle**.
- In **A**, nerve fibers of the **internal capsule** coursing between elements of the basal ganglia and **thalamus**.
- In **A**, the **sphenoid sinus**, with its mucoperiosteal lining protruding through the cut edge of the sphenoid bone.
- In **A**, the **optic nerve** sectioned close to the optic canal.
- In **B**, the **maxillary sinus** appearing as a dark signal.
- In **B**, the **sphenoid sinus** with its perimeter outlined by a bright signal effected by its mucoperiosteal lining.
- In **B**, the **transverse cerebral fissure** (**sylvian fissure**) outlined by cerebrospinal fluid (CSF).

Clinical Notes

- With aging, cerebral parenchyma often atrophies and the sulci increase in size. The increase is detected by MR imaging.
- Basal ganglia lie inferior to the lateral ventricle on sagittal sections and hemorrhage or lacunar infarction is well delineated in MR images.

References: G 7–1, 7–118 (excellent exposition of paranasal sinuses); RY 84, 88–89, schematic on 104, and see 108, 135

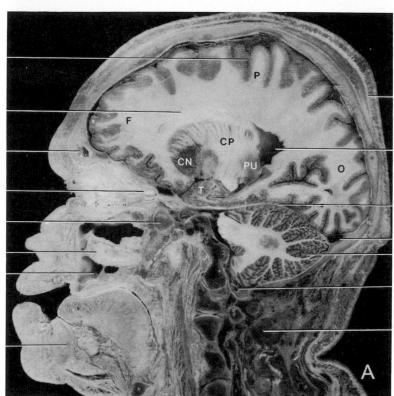

Central sulcus

Trunk of corpus callosum

Frontal sinus

Optic nerve

Sphenoid sinus

Middle nasal concha

Nasal cavity

Mandible

P

F

CP

CN

PU

O

T

Epicranial aponeurosis

Posterior horn of lateral ventricle

Tentorium cerebelli

Transverse sinus
Cerebellum

Vertebral artery

Spine of second cervical vertebra

A

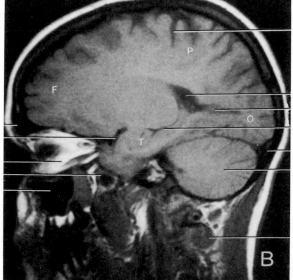

Central sulcus

Frontal sinus
Transverse cerebral fissure

Periorbital fat
Sphenoid sinus
Maxillary sinus

P

F

T

O

Body of lateral ventricle
Posterior horn of lateral ventricle
Temporal horn of lateral ventricle

Transverse sinus
Cerebellum

Spine of second cervical vertebra

B

CN-caudate nucleus **O**-occipital lobe **PU**-pulvinar
CP-internal capsule **P**-parietal lobe **T**-temporal lobe
F-frontal lobe

PLATE 15. Sagittal section through the nasal septum, hypophyseal fossa, and the tonsil of the cerebellum, T1 MR image

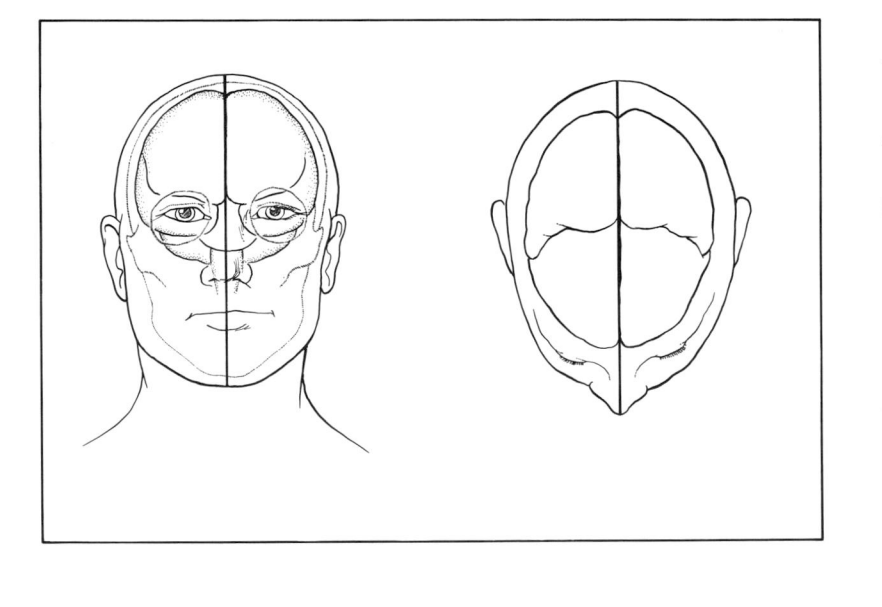

Note

- The **frontal** (*F*), **parietal** (*P*), and **occipital** (*O*) lobes of the cerebrum whose sulci in **B** are outlined by cerebrospinal fluid (CSF).
- Cranial to the cervical **spinal cord** (*SC*), the **medulla oblongata** (*MO*), the **pons** (*PO*), mesencephalon (*M*), and **diencephalon** (*D*).
- The **genu** (*g*), **trunk** (*tr*), and **splenium** (*s*) of the **corpus callosum**.
- Caudal to the **cerebellum**, the **cerebellomedullary cistern** (**cisterna magna**).
- The cavity and walls of the **fourth ventricle** outlined by cerebrospinal fluid (CSF) in **B**.
- The cerebral aqueduct passing through the **mesencephalon** from the third to the fourth ventricle.
- The **premedullary cistern** (*PC*) and the **foramen magnum** (*dashed line*).
- The **optic chiasma** superior to the **hypophyseal fossa** and the **pituitary gland** (**hypophysis**).
- The **caudate nucleus**, forming the lateral wall of the **body** of the cavity of the **lateral ventricle** in **A**, and the ventricle itself outlined by cerebrospinal fluid (CSF) in **B**.
- In **A**, the **tonsil** and **vermis** of the cerebellum.

Clinical Notes

- Midline sagittal MR imaging is excellent for visualization of pituitary tumors, which may extend superiorly and impinge on the optic chiasma or inferiorly to the sphenoid sinus.
- The cervicomedullary junction is surrounded by the premedullary cistern and the cisterna magna and may be compressed from bone disease, tumors, or tonsillar herniation due to elevated intracranial pressure from hemorrhage of cerebral or meningeal vessels.

References: G 7–1; RY 84

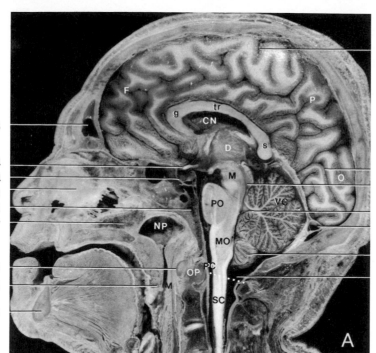

Central sulcus

Frontal sinus

Optic chiasma
Hypophyseal fossa
Nasal septum
Clivus
Vomer

Calcarine fissure
Cerebral aqueduct

Fourth ventricle
Transverse sinus

Anterior arch of atlas
Uvula

Tonsil of cerebellum
Cerebellomedullary cistern

Symphysis of mandible

A

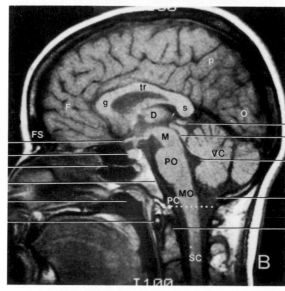

Optic chiasma
Hypophysis
Sphenoid sinus
Clivus
Nasopharynx
Anterior arch of atlas

Pineal gland
Cerebral aqueduct

Fourth ventricle

Cerebellomedullary cistern

Odontoid process

B

CN-caudate nucleus
D-diencephalon
F-frontal lobe
FS-frontal sinus

g-genu of corpus callosum
M-mesencephalon
MO-medulla oblongata
NP-nasopharynx

O-occipital lobe
OP-odontoid process
P-parietal lobe
PC-premedullary cistern

PO-pons
s-splenium of corpus callosum
SC-cervical spinal cord

tr-trunk of corpus callosum
VC-vermis of cerebellum
White dots-cisterna magna

PLATE 16. Sagittal head sections T1 MR image review

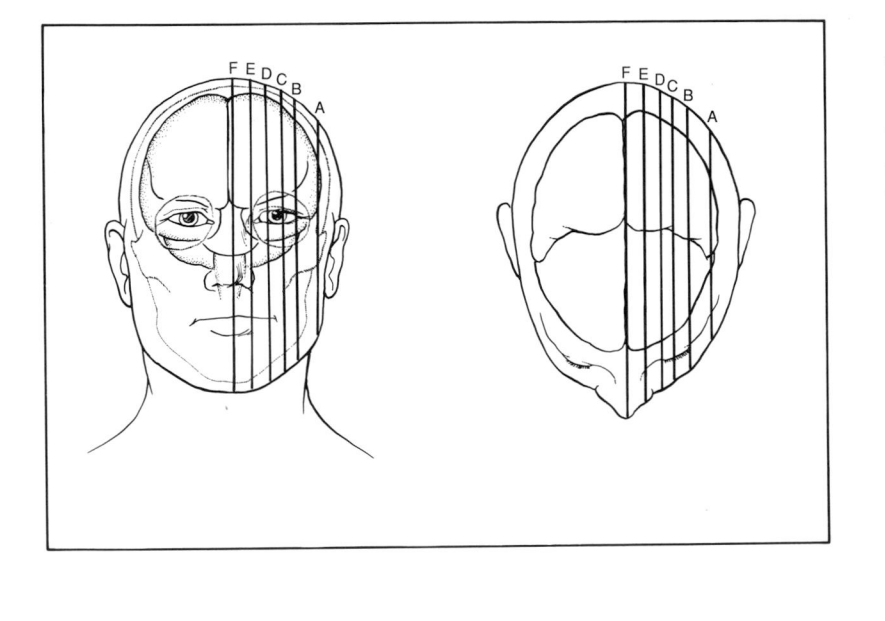

Note

A review of the plate below emphasizes how sectional anatomy can be used as a means for learning structural relationships. Referring to this plate and to previous ones, it is possible to trace the changing form and extent of different structures in a lateral to medial progression. While it is not feasible to describe each structure that appears, several examples can be listed.

Paranasal Sinuses

A, **B**, and **C** show the **maxillary sinus** (*MS*) in three different planes, **D** and **E** the **ethmoid sinus** (*ES*), and **E** and **F** the **sphenoid sinus** (*SS*).

Mandible and Infratemporal Region

A, **B**, and **C** show different parts of the mandible and muscle relationships to it: in **A**, the temporalis inserting into the coronoid process and the masseter on the angle of the mandible; **B** shows the medial side of the mandible with the medial pterygoid and superior to it the lateral pterygoid, while **C** shows the greater extent of the medial pterygoid.

Cranial Fossae

The relationship of the various lobes of the cerebrum (frontal, temporal) to the anterior and middle cranial fossae and the cerebellum to the posterior cranial fossa becomes apparent. The location of the brainstem, posterior to the clivus of the sphenoid and occipital bones, is also apparent.

Ventricular System and Cisterns

Each of the different parts of the lateral ventricles can be traced in images **B** to **F** (and in **E** and **F**, the fourth ventricle). In **F**, the cerebral aqueduct is visible as a midline structure. The cisterna magna is also clearly visualized.

Clinical Notes

In clinical evaluation, size, extent, relationship, and relative tissue characteristics of organs are all important diagnostic considerations. In practice, sequential MR or CT images are reviewed in sequences such as the sagittal sequence presented here. By referring to a series of images such as this, organs or structures are visualized through their extent. An orthogonal sequence, combining sagittal images with coronal or transaxial images, further aids visualization of the structure or lesion (abnormality) in its third dimension.

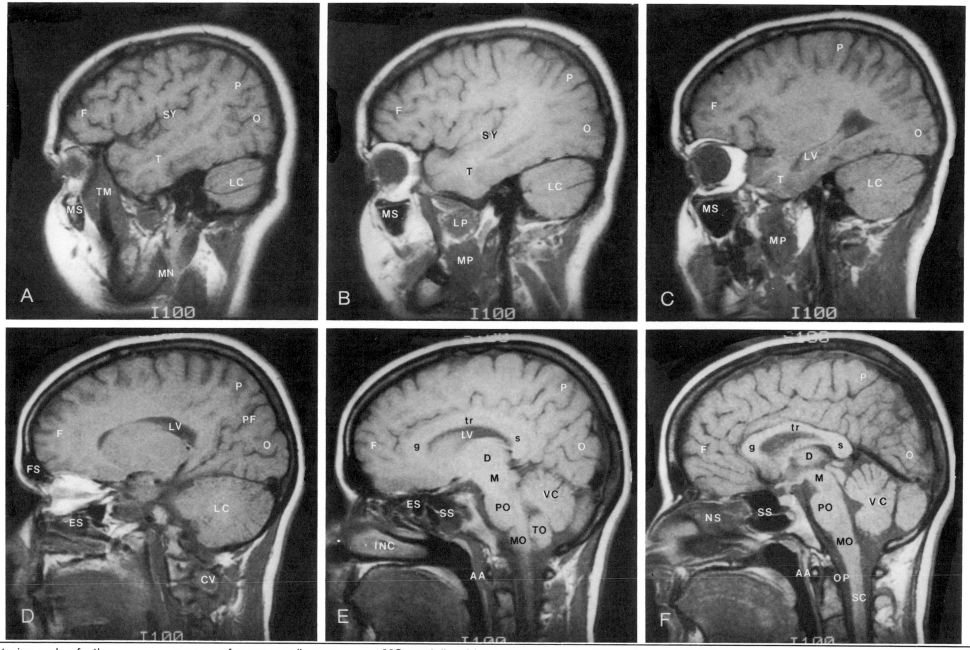

AA-anterior arch of atlas	**g**-genu of corpus callosum	**MO**-medulla oblongata	**PF**-parietooccipital fissure	**SY**-transverse cerebral fissure
CV-spine of second cervical vertebra	**INC**-inferior nasal concha	**MP**-medial pterygoid	**P**-parietal lobe	**T**-temporal lobe
D-diencephalon	**LC**-lateral lobe of cerebellum	**MS**-maxillary sinus	**PO**-pons	**TO**-tonsil of cerebellum
ES-ethmoid sinus	**LP**-lateral pterygoid	**NS**-nasal septum	**s**-splenium of corpus callosum	**TM**-temporalis
FS-frontal sinus	**LV**-cavity of lateral ventricle	**O**-occipital lobe	**SC**-spinal cord	**tr**-trunk of corpus callosum
F-frontal lobe	**M**-mesencephalon	**OP**-odontoid process	**SS**-sphenoid sinus	**VC**-vermis of cerebellum
	MN-mandible			

PLATE 20. Coronal section through corpus callosum, initial segment of mesencephalon, and oral cavity, T2 MR image

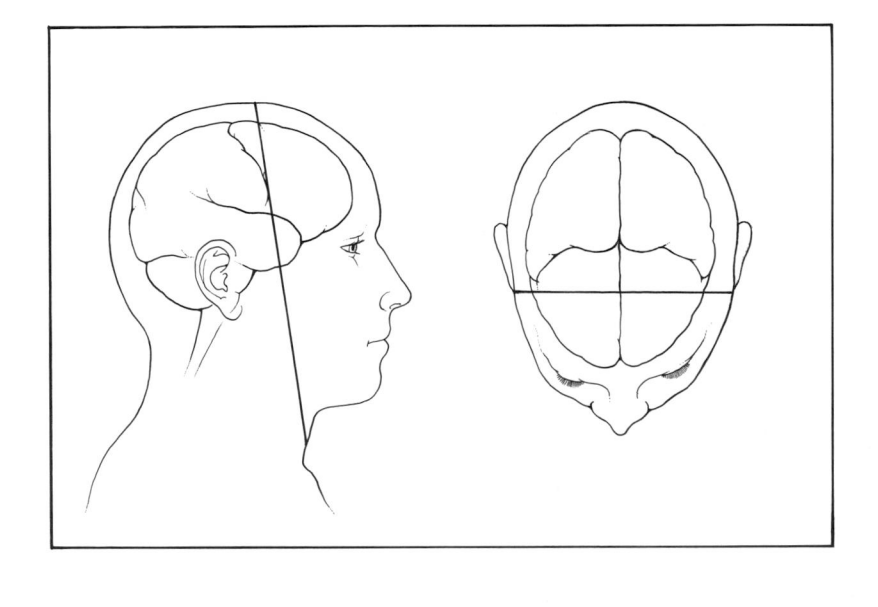

Note

- The **frontal** (*F*), **insular** (*I*), and **temporal** (*T*) lobes of the cerebrum.
- The **nasopharynx** inferior to the **sphenoid sinus**.
- The **superior sagittal sinus** and, extending inferiorly from it, the **falx cerebri**.
- The **sphenoid sinus**, outside whose lateral walls lies the **internal carotid artery** (*IC*) as it passes through the **cavernous sinus**.
- In **A**, the **trunk** (**body**) of the cavity of the **lateral ventricle** whose medial portion is bounded medially by the **fornix** (*f*).
- In **A**, the **temporal horn** of the cavity of the **lateral ventricle** adjacent to the **hippocampus**.

Clinical Notes

- The venous sinuses are demonstrated noninvasively by MR imaging.
- Venous thrombosis can occur in hypercoagulable states, such as those found in the postpartum patient. The degree of venous invasion is important in planning resection of adjacent meningiomas.
- Cavernous sinus thrombosis is less common than superior sagittal sinus thrombosis, which itself is uncommon.

References: G 7–25; 7–26; RY 85

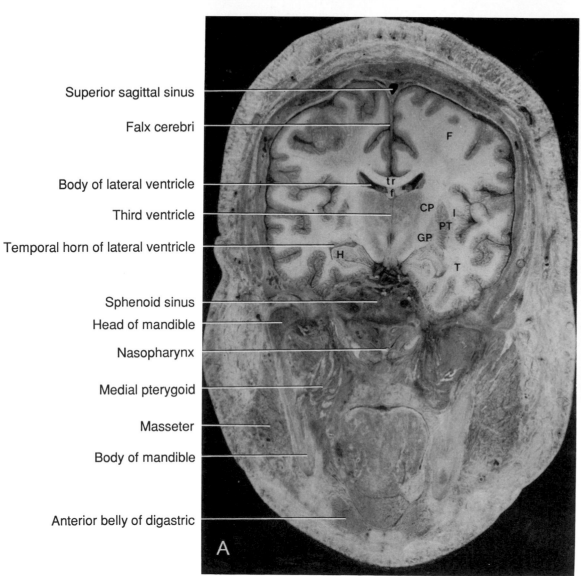

Superior sagittal sinus

Falx cerebri

Body of lateral ventricle

Third ventricle

Temporal horn of lateral ventricle

Sphenoid sinus

Head of mandible

Nasopharynx

Medial pterygoid

Masseter

Body of mandible

Anterior belly of digastric

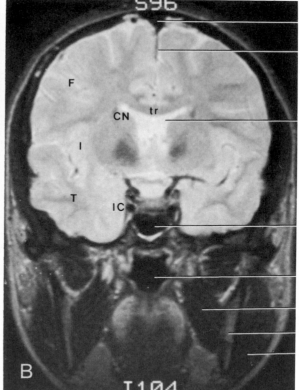

Superior sagittal sinus

Falx cerebri

Body of lateral ventricle

Sphenoid sinus

Nasopharynx

Medial pterygoid

Body of mandible

Masseter

CP-internal capsule	**H**-hippocampus	**IC**-internal carotid artery	**tr**-trunk of corpus callosum
F-frontal lobe	**I**-insular lobe	**T**-temporal lobe	**f**-fornix
GP-globus pallidus			

PLATE 21. Coronal section through the occipital lobe, medulla, and mastoid air cells, T2 MR image

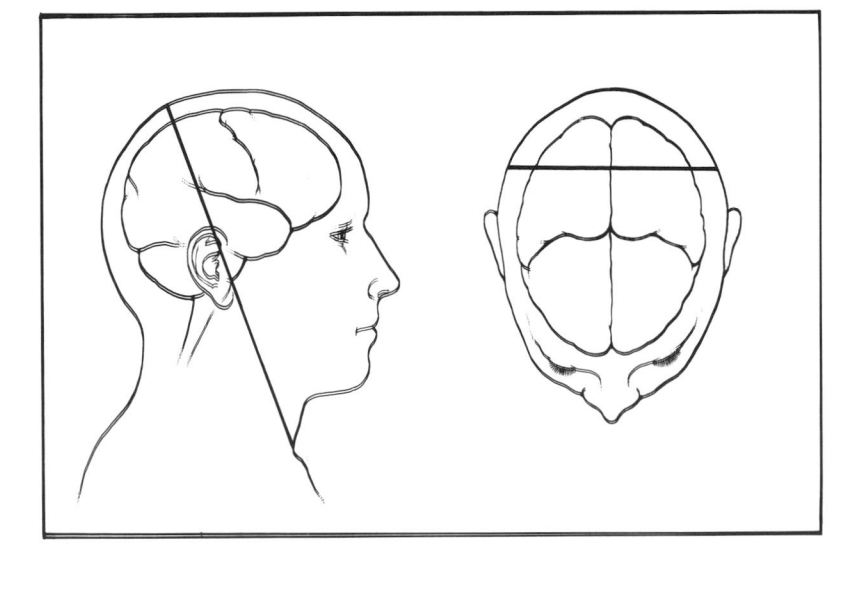

Note

- That **A** is cut at a somewhat more oblique angle than **B**.
- The **occipital lobe** (*O*), extending into which are the posterior horns of the **lateral ventricles**.
- The cavities of the **lateral ventricles**, outlined in **B** by cerebrospinal fluid (CSF).
- The **falx cerebri** extending from the **superior sagittal sinus** superiorly to the **inferior sagittal sinus** inferiorly.
- The **tentorium cerebelli** separating the cerebellum from the **occipital lobe** (*O*).
- The **parotid gland** inferior to the mastoid process with its contained **mastoid air cells**.
- In **A**, the **vermis** (*VC*) and **lateral lobes** (*LC*) of cerebellum.
- In **A**, the **fourth ventricle** and inferior to it the **medulla oblongata**.
- In **A**, the posterior part of the **cavity of the oropharynx**, showing the **uvula** (*UV*).

Clinical Notes

- Normal mastoid air cells are not delineated because of the low signal (*black*) from air and bone.

References: G 7–1, 7–32; RY 67 (almost identical posterior view), 84

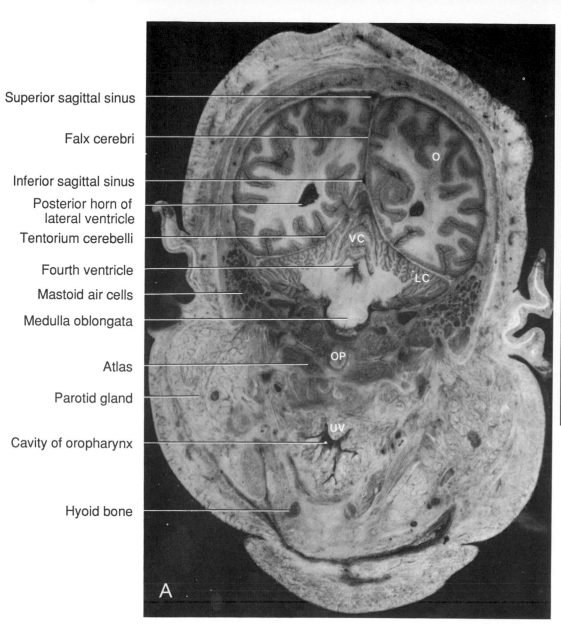

Superior sagittal sinus

Falx cerebri

Inferior sagittal sinus

Posterior horn of
lateral ventricle

Tentorium cerebelli

Fourth ventricle

Mastoid air cells

Medulla oblongata

Atlas

Parotid gland

Cavity of oropharynx

Hyoid bone

O

VC

LC

OP

UV

A

Superior sagittal sinus

Falx cerebri

Posterior horn of
lateral ventricle

Tentorium cerebelli

Mastoid air cells

Atlas

Axis

P

T

PO   LC

MO

OP

B

LC-lateral lobe of cerebellum   **OP**-odontoid process   **PO**-pons   **UV**-uvula
MO-medulla oblongata   **P**-parietal lobe   **T**-temporal lobe   **VC**-vermis of cerebellum
O-occipital lobe

PLATE 22. Coronal head T2 MR image review

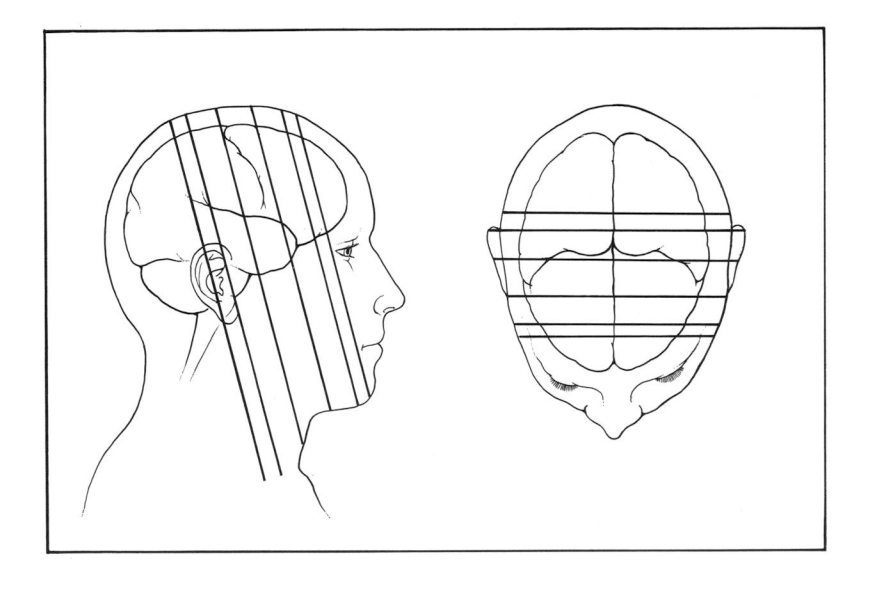

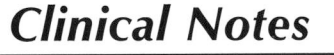

Note

As mentioned in the notes for the first review sequence (Plate 16), the analysis of sequential images, as in the coronal images in this plate, shows how sectional anatomy can be used to learn structural relationships. Cross-references between coronal, sagittal, and transaxial sections and images will enable the student to better conceptualize three-dimensional structure and relationships. As one example, the plate below shows the lateral ventricles through most of their anterior-to-posterior extent. The changing form of these structures at different levels can profitably be compared to preceding plates, which show views from superior to inferior and from lateral to medial.

Clinical Notes

See comment appearing with Plate 16, which also applies here.

References: Previous plates in this section.

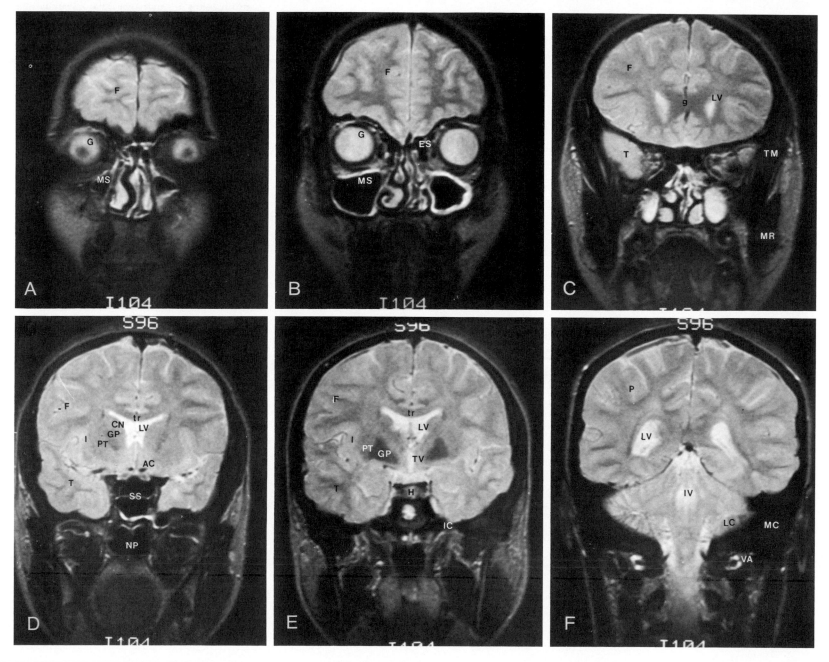

AC-anterior cerebral artery	**G**-globe	**IV**-fourth ventricle	**MR**-masseter	**T**-temporal lobe
CN-caudate nucleus	**GP**-globus pallidus	**LC**-lateral lobe of cerebellum	**NP**-nasopharynx	**tr**-trunk of corpus callosum
ES-ethmoid sinus	**H**-hypophysis (pituitary)	**LV**-lateral ventricle	**P**-parietal lobe	**TM**-temporalis
F-frontal lobe	**I**-insular lobe	**MC**-mastoid air cells	**PT**-putamen	**TV**-third ventricle
g-genu of corpus callosum	**IC**-internal carotid artery	**MS**-maxillary sinus	**SS**-sphenoid sinus	**VA**-vertebral artery

PLATE 23. Transaxial section through the clavicle, second part of the subclavian artery, and the dome of the pleura, T1 MR image

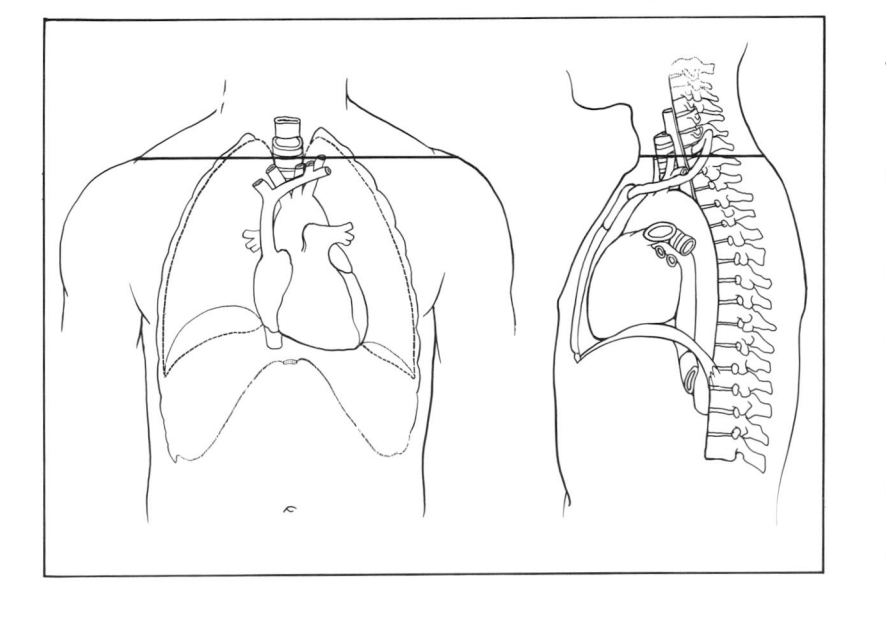

Note

- That **B** is inferior to **A**.
- The **spinal cord** surrounded by the subarachnoid space, which in **B** is outlined by cerebrospinal fluid (CSF).
- The **dura mater**, in **A**, external to which in **B** is the white signal of **epidural fat**.
- The **esophagus** (*E*), in **A** lying against the soft posterior wall of the **trachea** (*T*), and in **B** to its left side.
- The **internal jugular vein** (*IJ*) lateral to the **common carotid artery** and, in **A**, antero-lateral to the **vagus nerve**.
- In **A**, the **anterior scalene muscle** (*white dots*) and close to its medial side the **phrenic nerve**.
- In **A**, posterior to the **anterior scalene muscle, trunks of the brachial plexus** and, cut obliquely, the second part of the **subclavian artery**; medial to the **anterior scalene muscle** the first part of the **subclavian artery** with one of its branches, the **vertebral artery** (*VA*) on right.
- In **A**, the glistening **parietal pleura** at the pleural dome outlined here by parts of the **first rib**.
- In **B**, the long course of the **right brachiocephalic vein**, posterior to the **manubrium** of the sternum, heading toward the **superior vena cava.**
- In **B**, the anterior-to-posterior relationship of the **brachiocephalic, left common carotid**, and **left subclavian arteries**.

Clinical Notes

- The relationship of the pleural dome (hence pleural cavity) to the first rib explains why penetrating wounds in the lower region of the lateral neck can injure the lung.
- Trauma or intubation of the trachea may lead to tracheal stenosis, the degree of which is well evaluated by use of MR images in the transaxial, coronal, and sagittal planes.

References: G 1–48 (roof of the pleural cavity), 9–36, 9–37, 9–38, 9–46 (root of neck); RY 244–246, 249

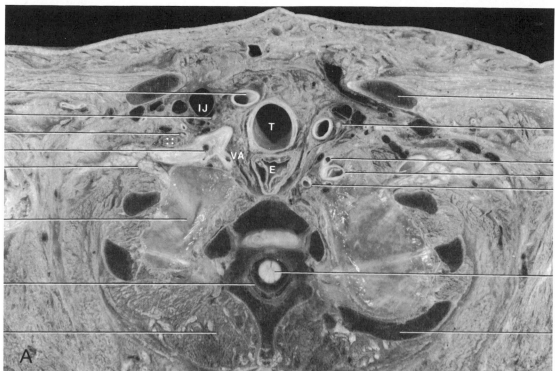

Common carotid artery

Vagus nerve

Phrenic nerve

Aditus of thyrocervical trunk

Lower trunks of brachial plexus

Dome of the parietal pleura

Dura mater

Semispinalis capitis

IJ

T

VA

E

Clavicle

Vagus nerve

Internal thoracic artery

Subclavian artery

Vertebral artery

Spinal cord

First rib

A

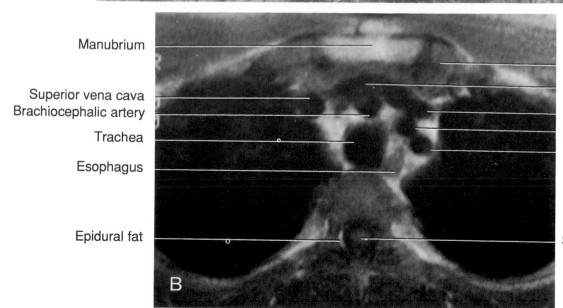

Manubrium

Superior vena cava

Brachiocephalic artery

Trachea

Esophagus

Epidural fat

Clavicle

Brachiocephalic vein

Subclavian vein

Common carotid artery

Subclavian artery

Spinal cord

B

E-esophagus   **T**-trachea   **White dots**-scalenus anterior

IJ-internal jugular vein   **VA**-vertebral artery

PLATE 24. Transaxial section through manubrium of sternum, arch of aorta, and body of fourth thoracic vertebra, T1 MR image

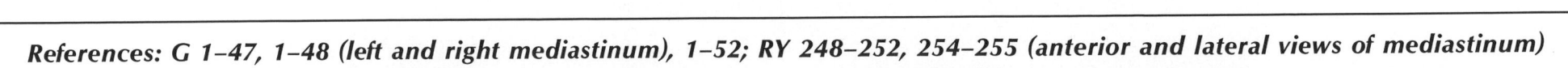

Note

- The anterior-to-posterior relationship of the **brachiocephalic**, **left common carotid**, and **left subclavian arteries** as they branch from the **arch of the aorta**.
- The **esophagus** posterior to the **trachea** (in **B**, e), often (as in this MR image) barely distinguishable due to normal contractions of its muscular walls which reduces the diameter of its lumen.
- The close approximation near the midline of the **upper lobes of the lung** separated from one another by **pleura** and **pericardial fat** which has extended superiorly from the heart to surround the great vessels (see Plates 25 and 26).
- In **A**, the **internal thoracic vessels**, seen through the **parietal pleura**.
- In **A**, the **azygos vein** posterior to the **esophagus**.
- In **A**, a large, pretracheal **lymph node** between the **superior vena cava** and the **trachea**.
- In **B**, the **superior vena cava** at the junction of the right and left brachiocephalic veins.

Clinical Notes

- Free-flowing blood generally gives a low-intensity signal (*dark*) within the vessel, allowing separation of vessels from lymph nodes and other tissue density structures, which have intermediate or higher signal intensity (*light*).
- Coronal MR image sections (not shown) are used to best demonstrate dissecting aortic aneurysms.
- MR imaging is generally not used for evaluating lung disease, because signal generation from the relatively minimal amount of tissue present is too low.
- Thymomas, often occurring in patients with myasthenia gravis, are located in the anterior mediastinum in the area of retrosternal fat. They are often invisible on plain radiographs but are clearly seen on MR images.

References: G 1–47, 1–48 (left and right mediastinum), 1–52; RY 248–252, 254–255 (anterior and lateral views of mediastinum)

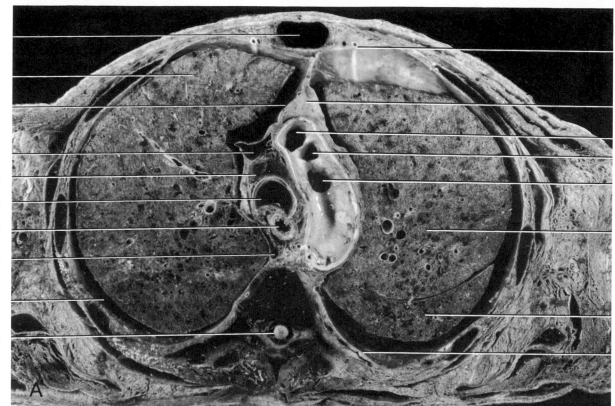

Sternum

Right upper lobe of lung

Mediastinal pleura

Superior vena cava

Pretracheal lymph node

Trachea

Esophagus

Azygos vein

Pleural cavity

Spinal cord

Internal thoracic artery

Pericardial fat

Brachiocephalic artery

Left common carotid artery

Left subclavian artery

Upper lobe of lung

Lower lobe of lung

Costal pleura

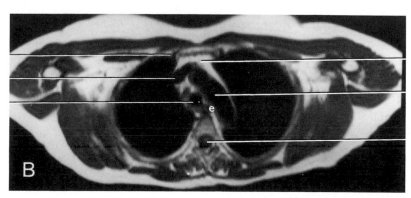

Internal thoracic artery

Superior vena cava

Trachea

Pericardial fat

Aortic arch

Spinal cord

e-esophagus

PLATE 25. Transaxial section at sternal angle through ascending aorta, tracheal bifurcation, and fourth thoracic vertebra, T1 MR image

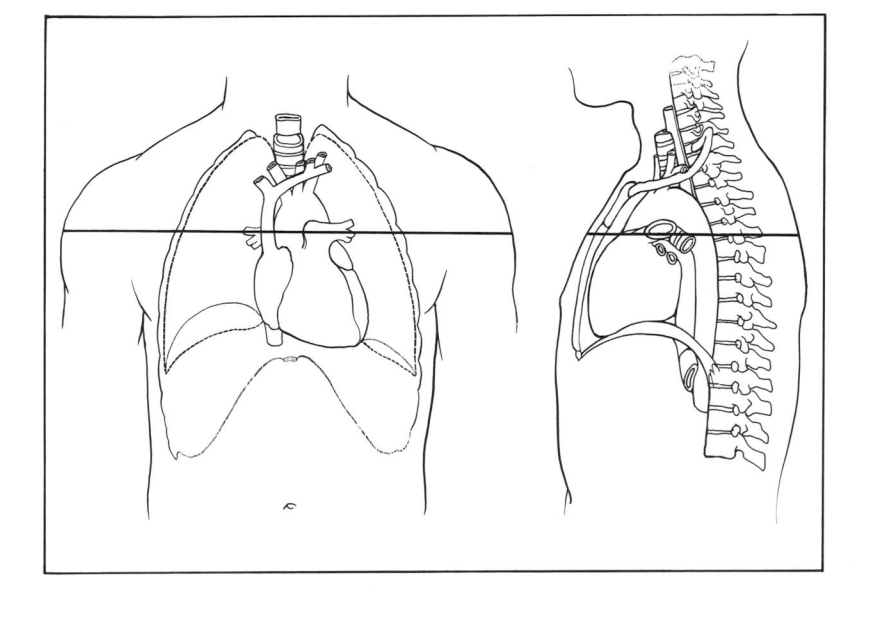

Note

- The costal cartilage of the **second rib** at the manubriosternal junction (sternal angle).
- The position of the **esophagus** (in **B**, *e*) posterior to the **left main bronchus**.
- The **ascending aorta** (in **B**, *aa*) to the left of the **superior vena cava**.
- The **left pulmonary artery** (in **B**, *lpa*) between the **ascending aorta** (in **B**, *aa*) and **descending aorta** (in **B**, *da*) and to the left of the **tracheal bifurcation** (in **A**, *tb*).
- In **A**, the **hemiazygos vein** posterior to the **descending aorta**.
- In **A**, the **azygos vein** posterior to the **esophagus** (in **B**, *e*).

Clinical Notes

- The aortopulmonary window (*apw*) and areas around the tracheal bifurcation are common sites for metastatic adenopathy.

References: G 1–47, 1–48 (left and right mediastinum), 1–79, 1–52 shows relations at tracheal bifurcation. RY 248–252, 254–255 (anterior and lateral views of mediastinum)

Second costal cartilage

Superior vena cava

Esophagus
Azygos vein

Body of fourth thoracic vertebra

Internal thoracic artery

Ascending aorta

Left pulmonary artery

Descending aorta

Hemiazygos vein

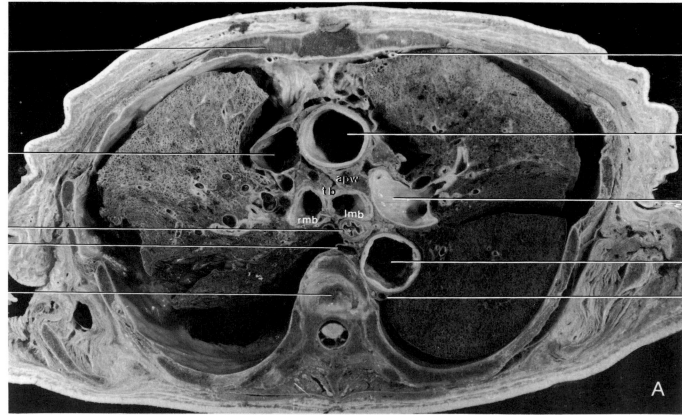

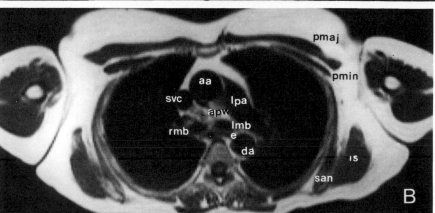

aa-ascending aorta
apw-aortopulmonary window
da-descending aorta

e-esophagus
is-infraspinatus
lmb-left main bronchus

lpa-left pulmonary artery
pmaj-pectoralis major
pmin-pectoralis minor

rmb-right main bronchus
san-serratus anterior

svc-superior vena cava
tb-tracheal bifurcation

PLATE 26. Transaxial section through sternum, ascending aorta, and right pulmonary artery, T1 MR image

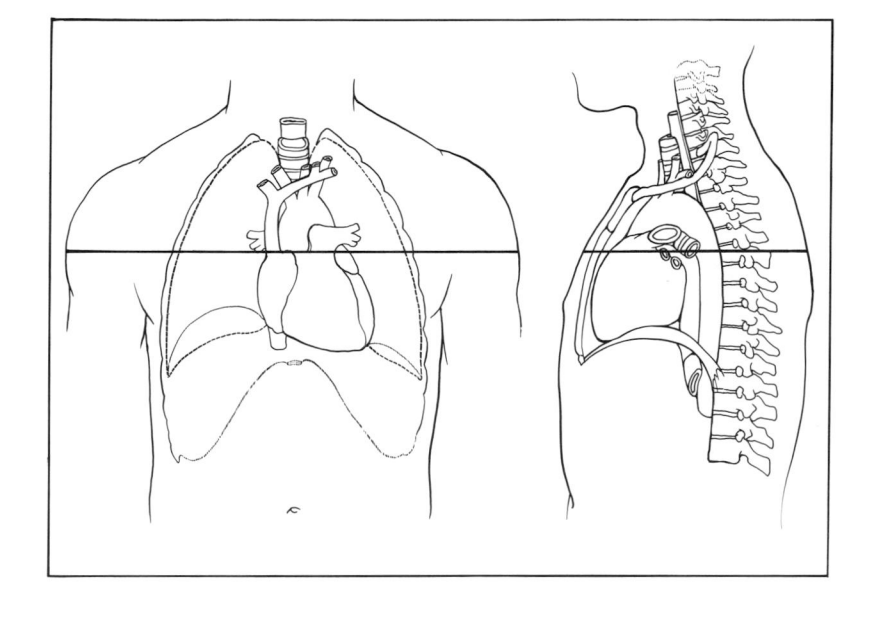

Note

- The **right** and **left main bronchi** (in **B**, *rmb*, *lmb*), with a branch of the left into the **left upper lobe bronchus** seen in **A**.
- The **ascending aorta** (in **B**, *aa*) medial to the **superior vena cava** (in **B**, *svc*) and anterior to the **right pulmonary artery** (in **B**, *rpa*).
- In **A**, the **esophagus** posterior to the left main bronchus and anterior to the **azygos vein**.
- In **A**, the **descending aorta** anterior to the **hemiazygos vein**.
- In **A**, the **pulmonary trunk** anterior to the **left main bronchus**.

Clinical Notes

- It is difficult to clearly visualize the esophagus on imaging studies because often, as here in **B**, it is collapsed (see page 47).
- The four most common anterior mediastinal lesions, which have the appearance of masses or disrupt the retrosternal fat, are thymomas, teratomas, substernal thyroids, and lymphomas.

References: G 1–47, 1–48 (left and right mediastinum), 1–52; RY 248–252, 254–255 (anterior and lateral views of mediastinum)

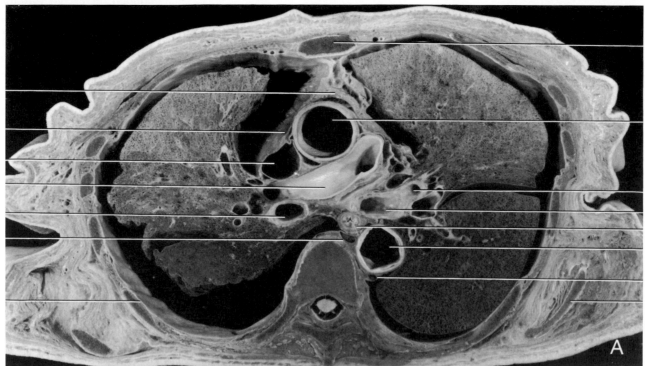

Pericardial fat

Mediastinal parietal pleura

Superior vena cava

Right pulmonary artery

Right main bronchus

Azygos vein

Costal parietal pleura

Body of sternum

Ascending aorta

Left upper lobe bronchus

Left main bronchus

Esophagus

Descending aorta

Hemiazygos vein

Scapula

A

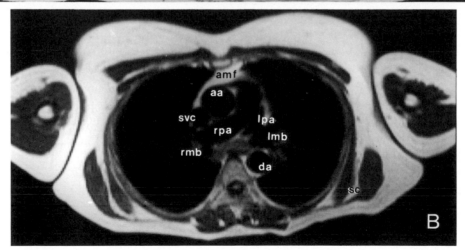

B

---

aa-ascending aorta   **lmb**-left main bronchus   **rmb**-right main bronchus   **sc**-scapula
amf-pericardial fat   **lpa**-left pulmonary artery   **rpa**-right pulmonary artery   **svc**-superior vena cava
da-descending aorta

PLATE 27. Transaxial section through sternum, left auricular appendage, and right pulmonary artery, T1 MR image

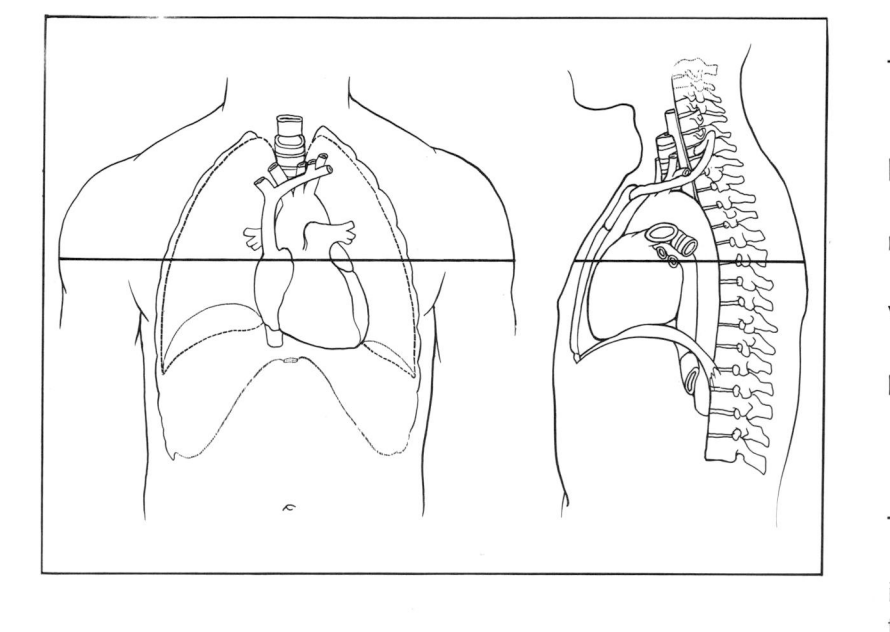

Note

- In **A**, the **right** and **left main bronchi**.
- Unlabeled, but occupying the space between and inferior to the **right** and **left main bronchi**, the clinically important **subcarinal space**.
- The **ascending aorta** (in **B**, *aa*) between the **superior vena cava** (in **B**, *svc*) and the **right pulmonary artery** (in **B**, *pa*).
- In **A**, the **esophagus** posterior to a **left pulmonary vein** and anterior to the **azygos vein**.
- In **A**, a reflection of **mediastinal parietal pleura** continuing with the **costal parietal pleura**, demonstrating that the **right** and **left pleural cavities** are separate from one another.
- In **A**, the **left auricle**, posterior to the **pulmonary arterial trunk**.

Clinical Notes

- Because the left atrial contour occupies the subcarinal space (see Plates 28 and 29) it is sometimes difficult to distinguish left atrial enlargement on CT scans. MR with multiplanar imaging of the flow void phenomenon is ideal to separate flowing blood (**dark signal**) from other tissue densities (**brighter signals**).

References: G 1–47, 1–48 (left and right mediastinum), 1–52; RY 248–252, 254–255 (anterior and lateral views of mediastinum)

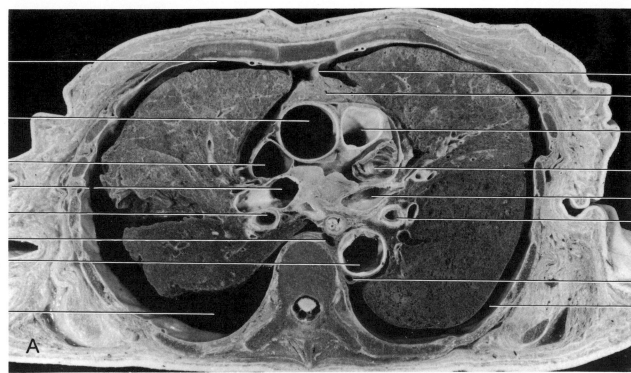

Costal parietal pleura

Ascending aorta

Superior vena cava

Right pulmonary artery

Right main bronchus

Azygos vein

Descending aorta

Pleural cavity

Mediastinal pleura

Pericardial fat

Trunk of pulmonary artery

Left auricle

Left pulmonary vein

Left main bronchus

Hemiazygos vein

Pleural cavity

A

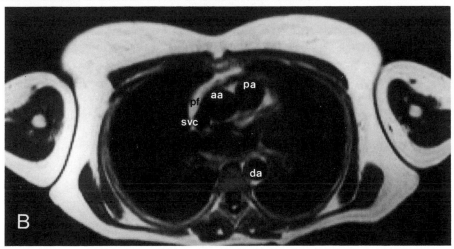

B

aa-ascending aorta   **e**-esophagus   **pf**-pericardial fat
da-descending aorta   **pa**-pulmonary artery   **svc**-superior vena cava

PLATE 28. Transaxial section through the sternum, base of heart, and descending aorta, T1 MR image

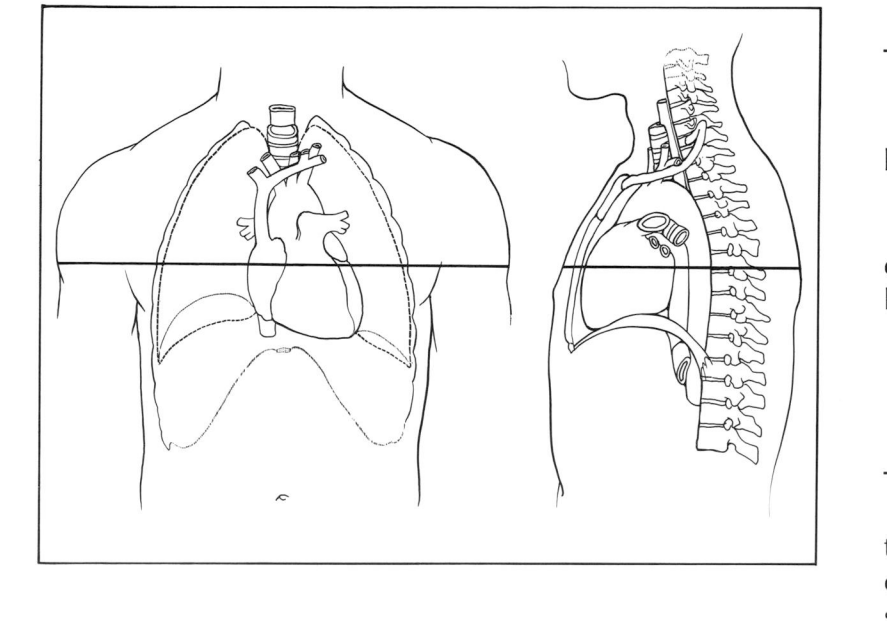

Note

- The root of the **ascending aorta** (in **B**, *aa*) anterior to the **left atrium** (in **B**, *la*).
- The **descending aorta** (in **B**, *da*) posterolateral to the **esophagus** and to the anterolateral side of the vertebral body.
- The **hemiazygos vein** (in **B**, *hav*) posterior to the **descending aorta** (in **B**, *da*).
- In **A**, the **right** and **left upper and lower lobes** of both lungs, with the right lung deflected laterally to more clearly reveal the **fibrous pericardium** against the black background.
- In **A**, the **cavity of the right atrium** near the level of the right atrioventricular valve.
- In **A**, the **esophagus** and its important posterior relationship to the **left atrium**.

Clinical Notes

- In various types of heart disease, an enlarged left atrium will press posteriorly into the posterior mediastinum. This is often seen as an esophageal constriction or extrinsic indentation on the barium swallow x-ray examination, and is also visible in MR images and CT scans.
- The azygos and hemiazygos veins are seen approximately 90% of the time in MR images. Any other structures, usually of intermediate density, especially those greater than 7–10 mm in diameter, are usually considered to be abnormal lymph nodes.

References: G 1–47, 1–48 (left and right mediastinum), 1–52; RY 248–252, 254–255 (anterior and lateral views of mediastinum)

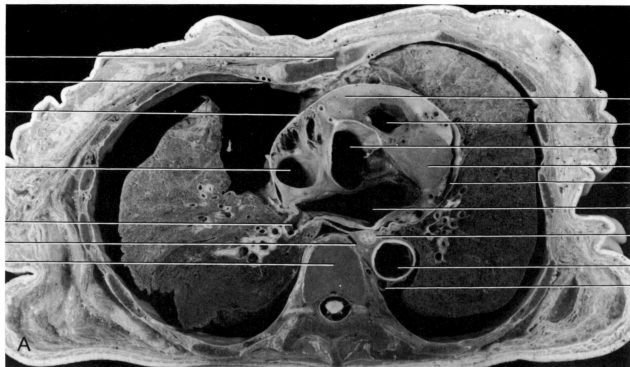

Sternocostal joint

Internal thoracic vessels

Fibrous pericardium

Cavity of right atrium

Pulmonary vein

Azygos vein

Vertebral body

Epicardial fat

Cavity of right ventricle

Ascending aorta

Myocardium of left ventricle

Pericardial cavity

Cavity of left atrium

Esophagus

Descending aorta

Hemiazygos vein

A

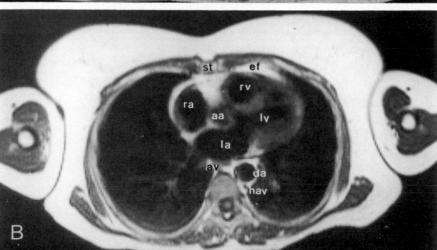

B

aa-ascending aorta	**da**-descending aorta	**hav**-hemiazygos vein	**lv**-left ventricle	**rv**-right ventricle
av-azygos vein	**ef**-epicardial fat	**la**-left atrium	**ra**-right atrium	**st**-sternum

PLATE 29. Transaxial section through the xiphoid process, left and right ventricles, and the tenth thoracic vertebra, T1 MR image

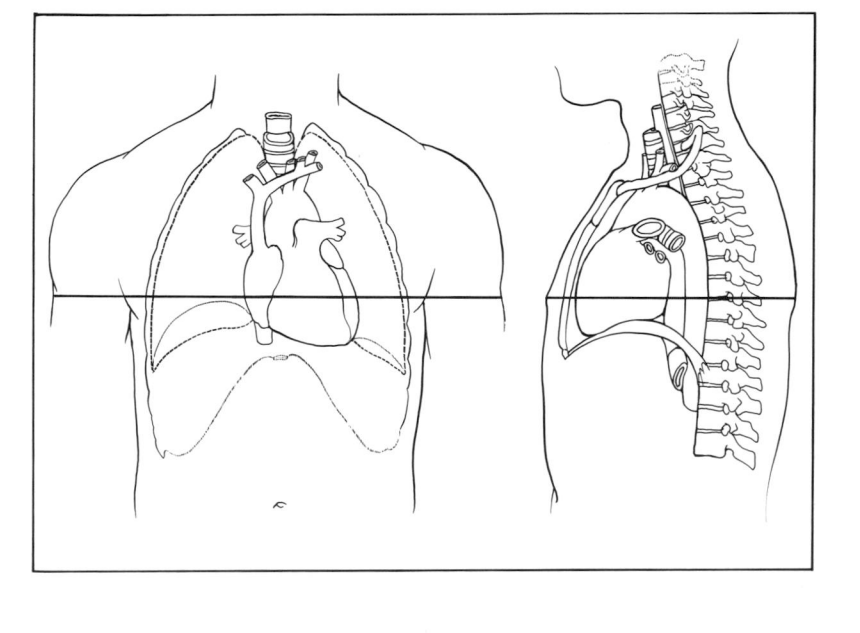

Note

- The **right atrium** (in **B**, *ra*) bulging slightly into the right pleural cavity.
- Superficial to the **fibrous pericardium** (in **B**, *p*), the **pericardial fat** (in **B**, *pf*).
- The thick **epicardial fat** (in **B**, *ef*) on the surface of the myocardium (a variable layer, see next comment).
- In **A**, the **pericardial cavity** between the **fibrous pericardium** and the **epicardium**, (visceral pericardium), here showing a thin layer of **epicardial fat**.
- The **esophagus** medial to the **descending aorta** and lateral to the **azygos vein**.
- The **hemiazygos vein** posterior to the **descending aorta**.
- In **A**, the thickness of the **left ventricular myocardium**, contrasting with that of the **right ventricular myocardium**.
- In **A**, the right lung deflected laterally to more clearly reveal the **fibrous pericardium** against the black background.

Clinical Notes

- Pericardial fat is coextensive with the fibrous pericardium, which extends superiorly and covers the beginnings of the great vessels and appears in this MR image. Note that pericardial fat is anatomically and clinically differentiated from the epicardial fat, which lies deep to the mesothelium of the visceral pericardium. The pericardial cavity, clinically most often a potential space, when enlarged, appears black and is well seen when contrasted between the pericardial and epicardial fat.
- Both the thin right atrial wall and the right ventricular wall contrast sharply with that of the left ventricle. Dynamic MR imaging (i.e., images obtained during specific phases of the cardiac cycle) is currently being investigated for the evaluation of cardiac function.

References: G 1–47, 1–48 (left and right mediastinum), 1–52; RY 248–252, 254–255 (anterior and lateral views of mediastinum)

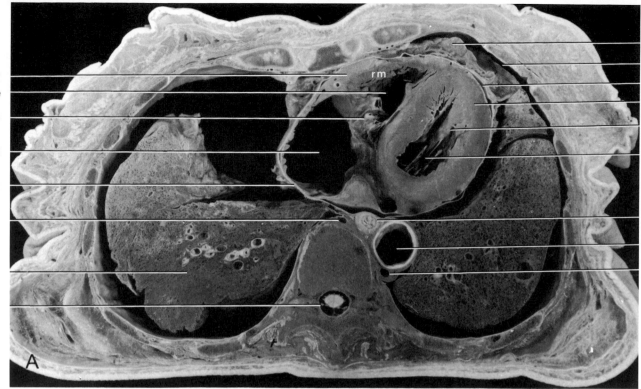

Epicardial fat
Cavity of right ventricle

Right atrioventricular valve

Cavity of right atrium

Fibrous pericardium

Azygos vein

Right lower lobe of lung

Thoracic spinal cord

Pericardial fat
Pleural cavity
Pericardial cavity
Myocardium of left ventricle
Papillary muscle

Chordae tendineae

Esophagus

Descending aorta

Hemiazygos vein

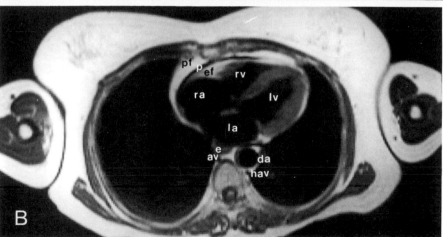

av-azygos vein
da-descending aorta
e-esophagus

ef-epicardial fat
hav-hemiazygos vein
la-left atrium

lv-left ventricle
p-fibrous pericardium

pf-pericardial fat
ra-right atrium

rm-right ventricular myocardium
rv-right ventricle

PLATE 30. Transaxial section of costodiaphragmatic region of the lungs, right lobe of the liver, and pericardial cavity, T1 MR image

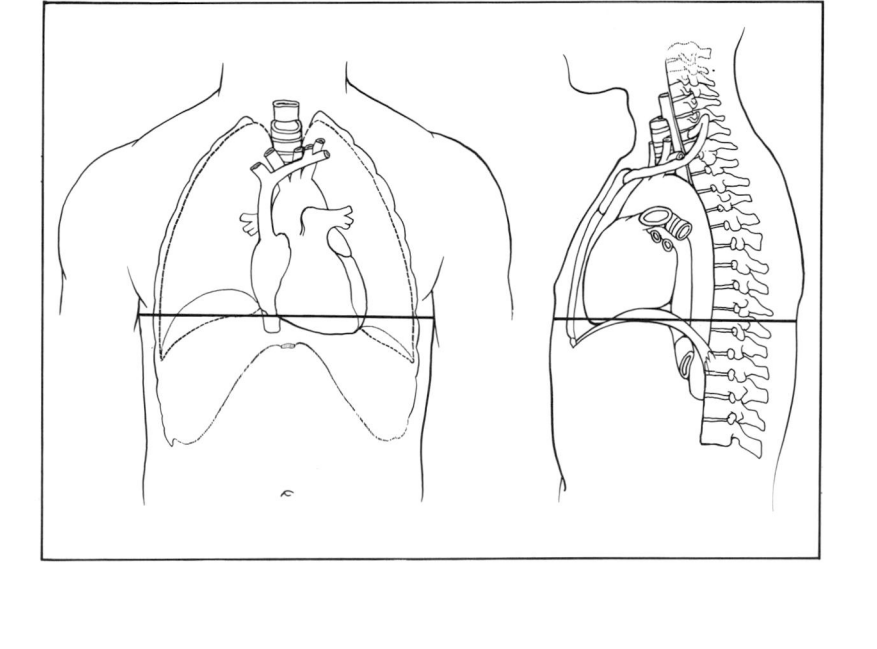

Note

- That **A** is slightly superior to **B**.
- The region near the **apex** of the **heart** seen through the cut edges of the **fibrous pericardium** in **A** and covered by a glistening layer of the epicardium (visceral pericardium).
- The **right** (in **A**, *RH*) and **left** (in **A**, *LH*) **hepatic veins** entering the **inferior vena cava** (*IVC*).
- The **cardiac portion of the stomach** lying just anterior to the **abdominal aorta**, which itself is just lateral to the **azygos vein** (*AV*).
- In **A**, the **right** and **left lower lobes** of the lungs and the **pleural cavity**.
- In **A**, the **right lobe of the liver** related to its right by the cut edges of the **diaphragm**; between liver and diaphragm a small portion of the **peritoneal cavity**.
- In **B**, the caudal extent of both the anterior pleural cavity and the posterior costophrenic sulcus.

Clinical Notes

- In various lung diseases, pleural fluid often fills the costophrenic spaces and is removed by thoracentesis (percutaneous needle aspiration). The proximity of the lung and the liver on the right, and the lung and spleen on the left shows how the liver, an abdominal organ, may easily be involved in attempts to remove fluid from the pleural cavity or in thoracic wall injury.
- MR imaging is extremely sensitive to motion artifacts from breathing and pulse artifacts from aortic and visceral movement (bowel peristalsis) because of the relatively long (3–17 minute) data acquisition times. Research is continuing toward the development of faster scan techniques to alleviate this problem.
- The normally thin diaphragm is poorly visualized by sectional imaging techniques such as MR and CT.
- Visualization of the flow void within the hepatic veins and hepatic vein confluence is crucial in excluding hepatic vein thrombosis (Budd-Chiari syndrome).
- The pleural fat, when more extensive, can mimic a pleural-based lesion, such as asbestosis, on plain radiographs.

References: G 2–27, 2–119; RY 25B

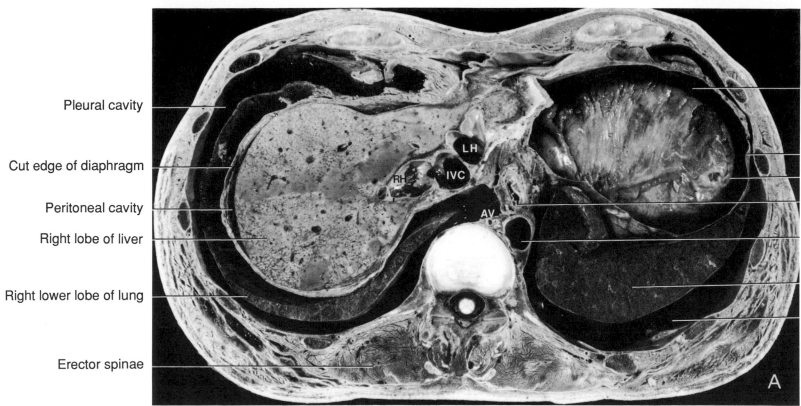

Pleural cavity

Cut edge of diaphragm

Peritoneal cavity

Right lobe of liver

Right lower lobe of lung

Erector spinae

Pericardial cavity

Fibrous pericardium

Apex of heart

Cardiac portion of stomach

Abdominal aorta

Left lower lobe of lung

Pleural cavity

LH

RH   IVC

AV

A

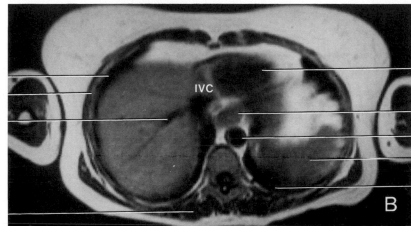

Peritoneal cavity
Diaphragm

Right hepatic vein

Erector spinae

IVC

Apex of heart

Cardiac part of stomach

Abdominal aorta

Spleen

Peritoneal cavity

B

AV-azygos vein   **IVC**-inferior vena cava
LH-left hepatic vein   **RH**-right hepatic vein

PLATE 31. Transaxial thorax T1 MR image review

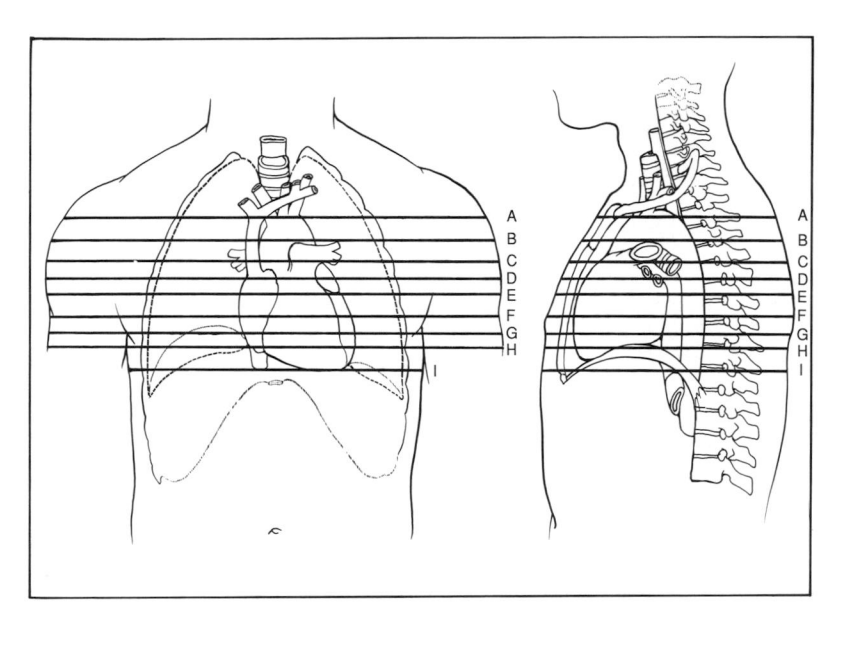

Note

A review of the plate below emphasizes the usefulness of multiple-image plates revealing, as mentioned in previous review plates, how sectional anatomy can be used as a means for learning structural relationships. Referring to this plate and to previous ones, it is possible to trace the form and extent of different structures in their anterior-to-posterior and superior-to-inferior course. This allows one to build a three-dimensional concept of the various structures and their relationships to one another.

Clinical Notes

Observing multiple images allows one to more certainly define the location and extent of structures or the degree to which pathological processes have involved a region. Sequential images are often necessary in the clinical setting because of anatomical variations in the course of longitudinally oriented structures.

References: Plates 17–30

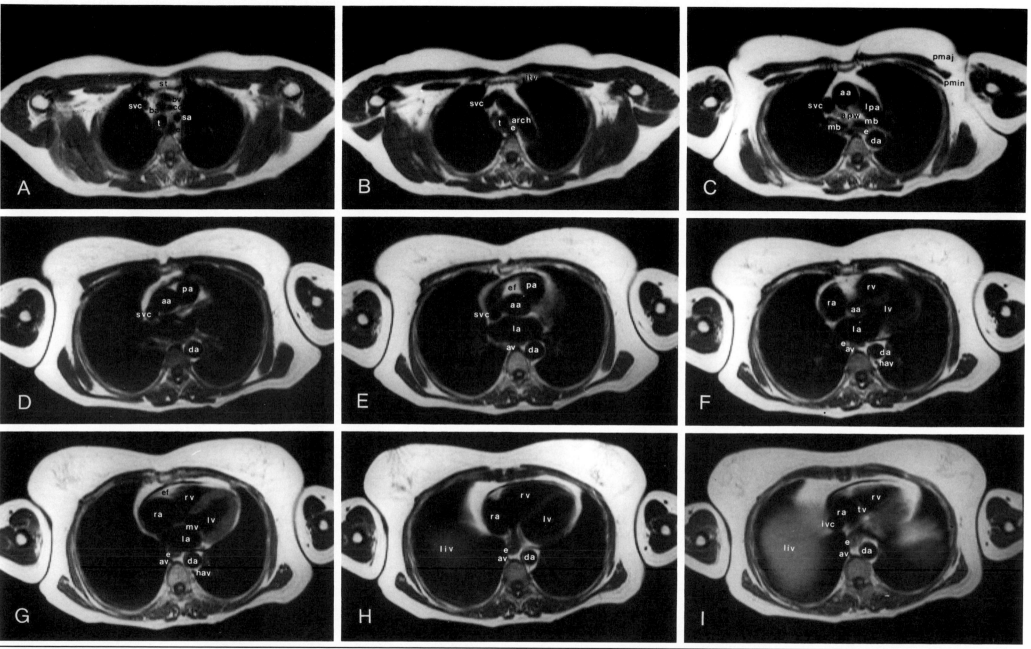

aa-ascending aorta
apw-aortopulmonary window
arch-arch of aorta
av-azygos vein
ba-brachiocephalic artery
bv-left brachiocephalic vein

cc-left common carotid artery
da-descending aorta
e-esophagus
ef-epicardial fat
hav-hemiazygos vein
itv-internal thoracic vessels

ivc-inferior vena cava
la-left atrium
lpa-left pulmonary artery
liv-liver
lv-cavity of left ventricle
mb-main bronchus

mv-bicuspid valve
pa-main pulmonary artery
pmaj-pectoralis major
pmin-pectoralis minor
ra-cavity of right atrium
rv-right ventricle

sa-subclavian artery (left)
st-sternum
svc-superior vena cava
t-trachea
tv-tricuspid valve

PLATE 32. Transaxial section through costodiaphragmatic recesses, liver at porta hepatis, and spleen, CT scan, oral iodinated contrast

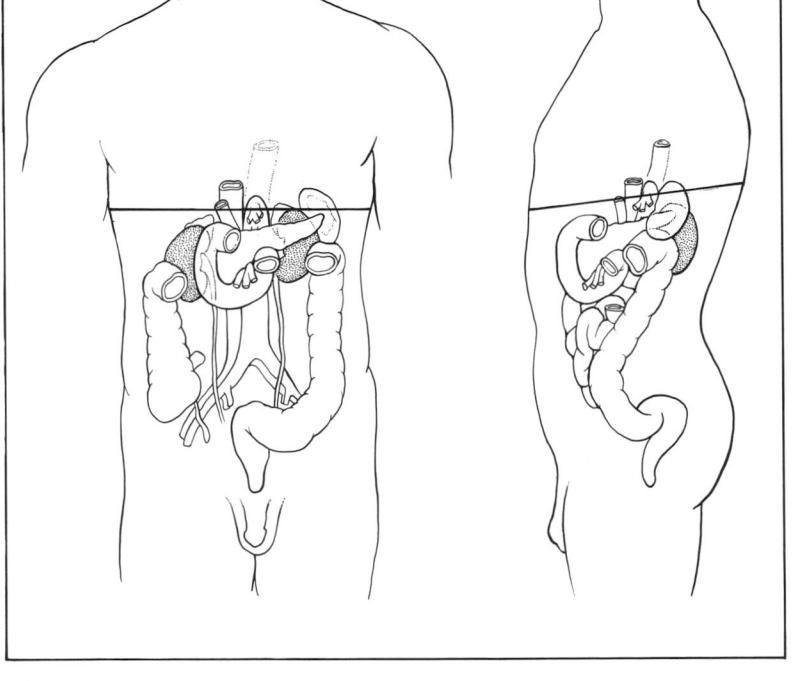

Note

- That **B** is slightly inferior to **A**, which is cut slightly obliquely, thus passing superior to the kidneys, as indicated in the diagram.
- The **right** and **left** lobes of the **liver**.
- The **peritoneal cavity** to the right of the **right lobe of the liver**.
- The right **adrenal gland** posterolateral to the **inferior vena cava** and medial to the **right lobe of liver** in **A**, and the left **adrenal gland** between the **body of the stomach** and the **abdominal aorta** in **B**.
- The posterior abdominal musculature, here represented by **psoas major** and **quadratus lumborum** muscles.
- The **spleen** posterior to the **body of the stomach**.
- The **inferior vena cava** just posterior to the **portal vein**.
- The **abdominal aorta** and the vessel just anterior to it, the **celiac artery**.
- In **A**, the cut edge of the **diaphragm**.
- In **A**, the **right** and **left costodiaphragmatic recesses** close to the inferiormost extent of the pleural cavity.
- In **A**, the **spinal cord** sectioned at the **conus medullaris** surrounded by the cauda equina and occupying the cranial limit of the lumbar cistern.

Clinical Notes

- Fat planes surrounding the celiac and superior mesenteric arteries are preferential sites for the spread of pancreatic cancer.
- The adrenal glands are often the site of metastasis from lung cancer, the demonstration of which usually makes the patient inoperable.
- Adrenal masses can be visualized using MR imaging. T2 tissue characteristics are often highly suspicious for malignancy, especially malignant pheochromocytoma.

References: G 2–28, 2–34, 2–72, 2–73, 2–85, 2–115; RY 293–295

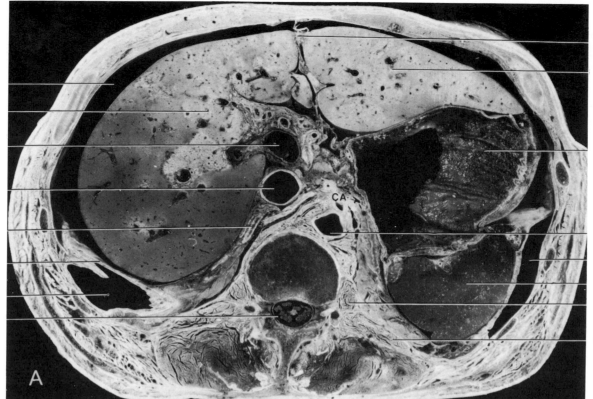

Peritoneal cavity

Right lobe of liver

Portal vein

Inferior vena cava

Adrenal gland

Cut edge of diaphragm

Costodiaphragmatic recess

Cauda equina

Falciform ligament

Left lobe of liver

Body of stomach

Abdominal aorta

Costodiaphragmatic recess

Spleen

Psoas major

Quadratus lumborum

CA

A

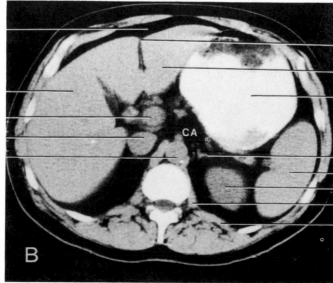

Peritoneal cavity

Right lobe of liver

Portal vein

Inferior vena cava

Abdominal aorta

Falciform ligament

Left lobe of liver

Body of stomach

Left adrenal gland

Spleen

Upper pole of kidney

Psoas major

Quadratus lumborum

CA

B

CA-celiac artery

PLATE 33. Transaxial section through left and right lobes of liver, spleen, and head of pancreas, CT scan, oral iodinated contrast

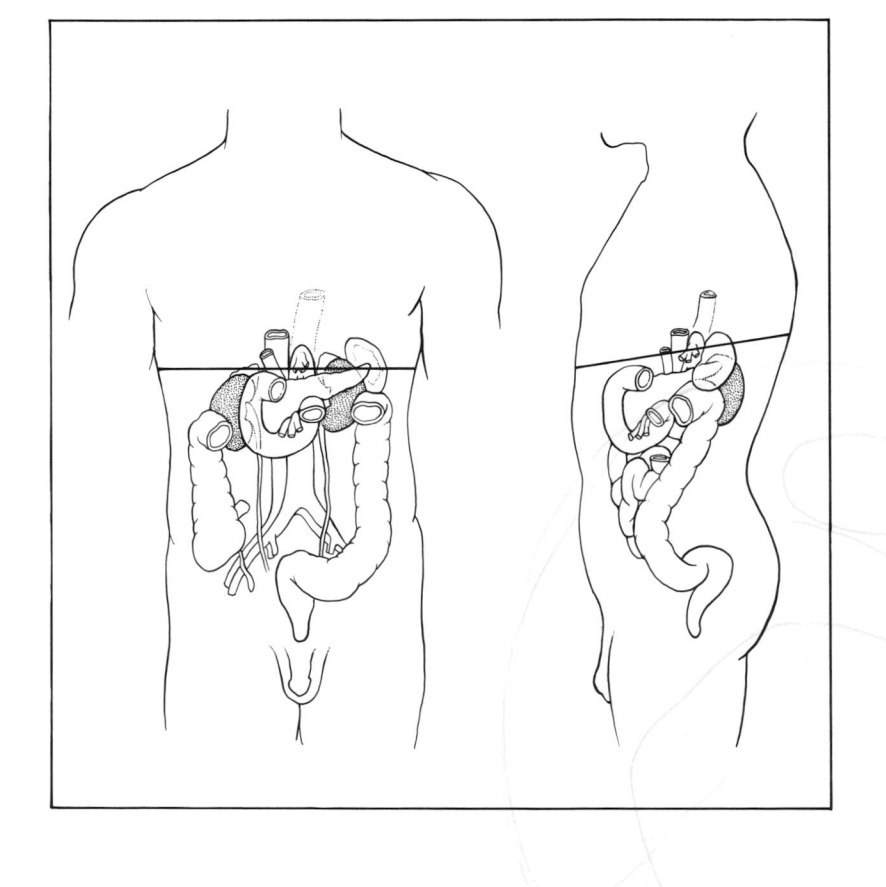

Note

- The **right** and **left lobes of the liver**, between which in **A** is the **first part** of the **duodenum** and, in **B**, the **second part** of the **duodenum**.
- Posterior to the **portal vein**, the **inferior vena cava**.
- The **spleen** and its anterior relationship, the **body of the stomach**.
- In **A**, anterolateral to the **duodenum**, the head of the **pancreas** and, partly embedded in the pancreas, the **portal vein**.
- In **A**, occupying the lumbar cistern in the spinal canal, the **cauda equina**.
- In **A**, the **perirenal fat**, embedded in which is the left **adrenal gland** between the **splenic vein** and the **abdominal aorta**.

Clinical Notes

- It is often impossible, without intravenous contrast, to differentiate the portal vein from the head of the pancreas.
- The falciform ligament separates the medial from the lateral segment of the left lobe of the liver.

References: G 2–28, 2–34, 2–72, 2–73, 2–85, 2–115; RY 293–295

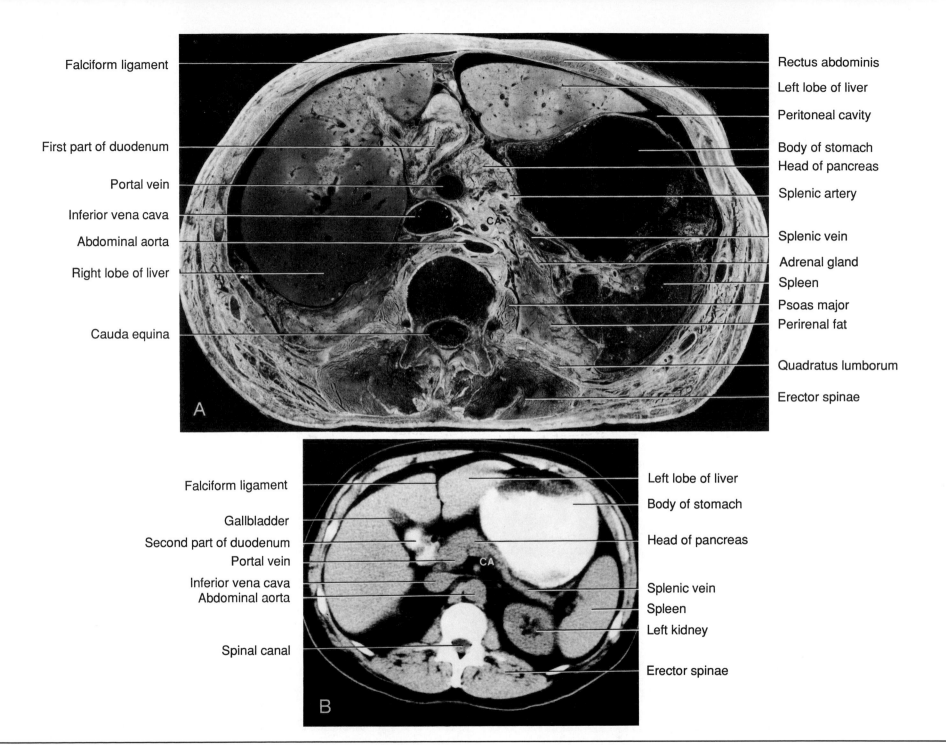

Falciform ligament

First part of duodenum

Portal vein

Inferior vena cava

Abdominal aorta

Right lobe of liver

Cauda equina

Rectus abdominis

Left lobe of liver

Peritoneal cavity

Body of stomach
Head of pancreas

Splenic artery

Splenic vein

Adrenal gland

Spleen

Psoas major

Perirenal fat

Quadratus lumborum

Erector spinae

A

Falciform ligament

Gallbladder

Second part of duodenum
Portal vein

Inferior vena cava
Abdominal aorta

Spinal canal

Left lobe of liver

Body of stomach

Head of pancreas

Splenic vein

Spleen

Left kidney

Erector spinae

B

CA-celiac artery

PLATE 34. Transaxial section through the right lobe of liver, gallbladder, and spleen, CT scan, oral iodinated contrast

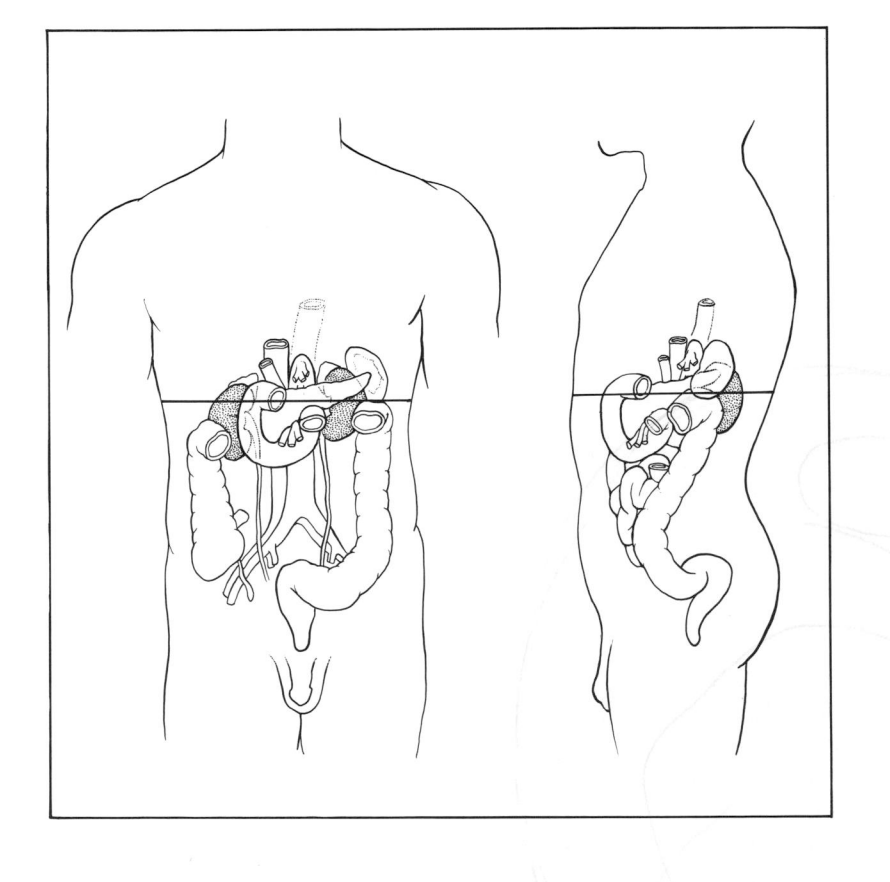

Note

- The **right** and **left lobes of the liver** and between them the **gallbladder**, and to its left the **pyloric antrum of the stomach**.
- The **descending part of the duodenum** and to its immediate left the **uncinate process**.
- The **body of the pancreas** extending laterally, posterior to the body of the **stomach**, its **tail** reaching as far as the **spleen**.
- The **superior poles** of both **kidneys** and portions of the **renal artery** and **renal vein** surrounded by copious **perirenal fat**.
- The **inferior vena cava** (*IVC*) lying nearly side-by-side with the **abdominal aorta** (*A*) and both vessels lying posterior to the body of the **pancreas**.
- In **A**, the **head** of the **pancreas** embedding the **superior mesenteric vein** and just posterior to this vein the **superior mesenteric artery**.
- In **A**, occupying the lumbar cistern in the spinal canal, the **cauda equina**.

Clinical Notes

- The superior mesenteric artery is anterior to the left renal vein and may compress it against the aorta, resulting in venous stasis.
- The oblique course of the pancreas usually results in the head, body, and tail being seen on different transaxial images. Imaging of pancreatic disease is currently best performed by CT or diagnostic ultrasound scanning.

References: G 2–28, 2–34, 2–72, 2–73, 2–85, 2–115; RY 293–295

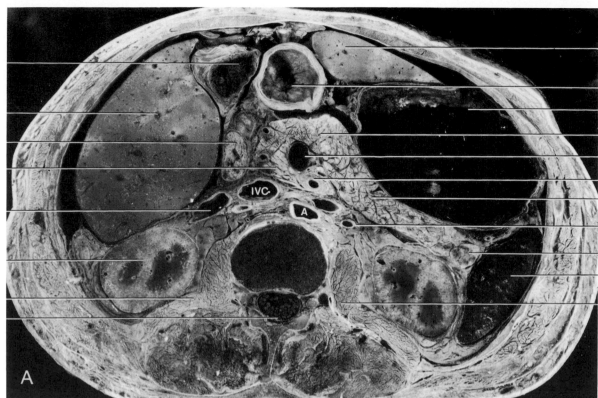

Gallbladder

Right lobe of liver

Second part of duodenum

Uncinate process of pancreas

Right renal vein

Right kidney

Quadratus lumborum
Cauda equina

Left lobe of liver

Pyloric antrum of stomach

Body of stomach

Head of pancreas

Superior mesenteric vein

Superior mesenteric artery

Body of pancreas

Left renal artery

Tail of pancreas

Spleen

Psoas major

IVC

A

A

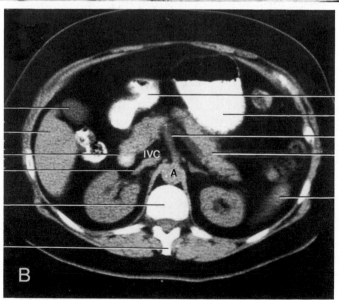

Gallbladder

Right lobe of liver

Second part of duodenum
Right renal vein

Vertebral body

Spinous process

Pyloric antrum of stomach

Body of stomach

Superior mesenteric artery

Body of pancreas

Spleen

IVC

A

B

A-abdominal aorta
IVC-inferior vena cava

PLATE 35. Transaxial section through the right lobe of the liver, hilum of kidneys, and spleen, CT scan, oral iodinated contrast

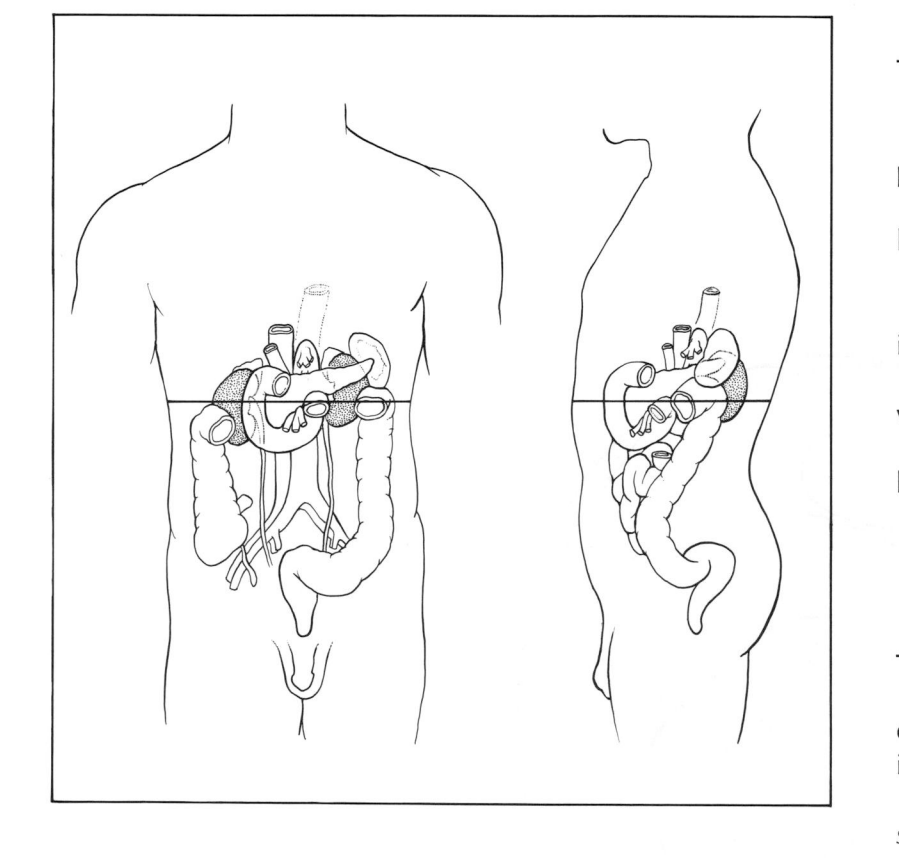

Note

- That **A** is slightly inferior to **B**.
- The **right lobe of the liver** in contact with the **transverse colon** to the right of the **pyloric antrum** of the stomach.
- The **second** or descending **part of the duodenum** abutting the **pancreas** and lying between it and two of the organs it contacts: the **right lobe of the liver** and the **right kidney**.
- The **renal pelvis** of the **right kidney.**
- In **A**, the **superior mesenteric artery** and **vein** in the substance of the **pancreas** and, in **B**, this same artery branching from the **abdominal aorta** (*A*) posterior to the pancreas.
- The **left renal vein** and, posterior to it, the **left renal artery** in **A** and the **right renal vein** in **B**.
- The **inferior vena cava** and the **abdominal aorta** lying side by side and both vessels lying posterior to the body of the **pancreas**.
- In **A**, the inferior tip of the **spleen**.
- In **A**, occupying the lumbar cistern in the spinal canal, the **cauda equina**.

Clinical Notes

- The ascending colon, the second part of the duodenum, the pancreas, and the descending colon all lie in contiguity in the anterior pararenal space. This relationship is important in evaluating the contiguous spread of disease.
- Pathological changes are well visualized in CT scans. Here, tiny calcifications (*white spots*) on the inner wall of the abdominal aorta appear, signaling arteriosclerotic change. Occasionally, the wall of the aorta develops weak spots, leading to ballooning (aneurysm formation). When the aorta measures more than 3.5 cm it is considered to be aneurysmal. Patients with aneurysms greater than 5.0 cm are candidates for surgery.

References: G 2–28, 2–34, 2–72, 2–73, 2–85, 2–115; RY 293–295

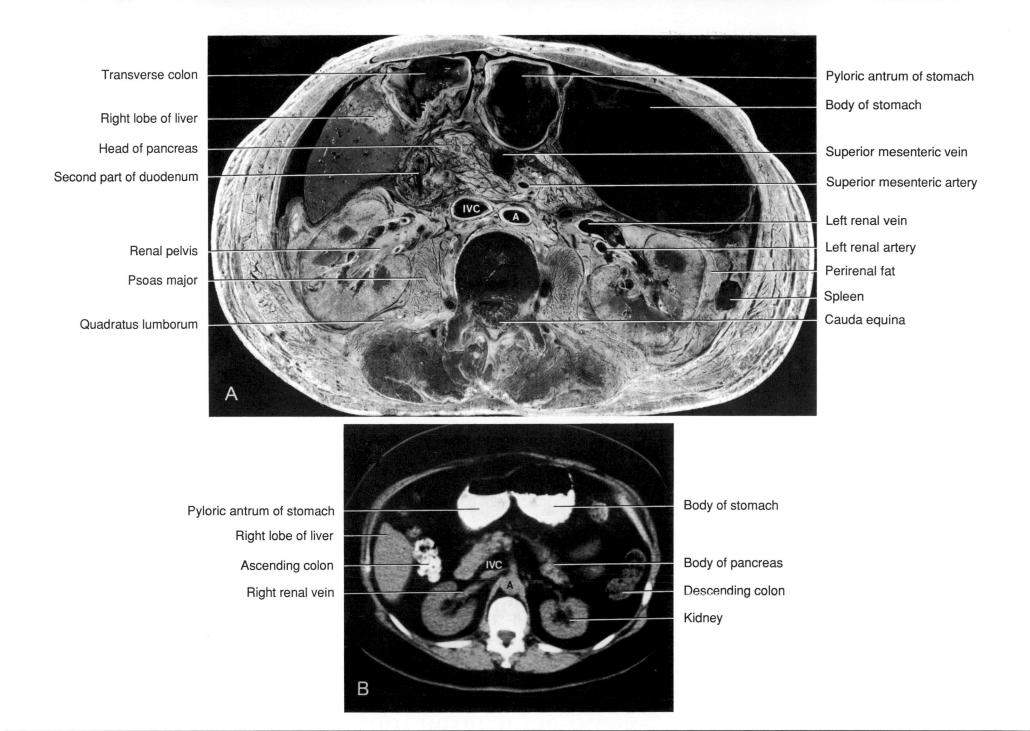

Transverse colon

Right lobe of liver

Head of pancreas

Second part of duodenum

Renal pelvis

Psoas major

Quadratus lumborum

Pyloric antrum of stomach

Body of stomach

Superior mesenteric vein

Superior mesenteric artery

Left renal vein

Left renal artery

Perirenal fat

Spleen

Cauda equina

IVC

A

A

Pyloric antrum of stomach

Right lobe of liver

Ascending colon

Right renal vein

Body of stomach

Body of pancreas

Descending colon

Kidney

IVC

A

B

A-abdominal aorta
IVC-inferior vena cava

PLATE 36. Transaxial section through the transverse duodenum, kidneys, and descending colon, CT scan, oral and intravenous iodinated contrast

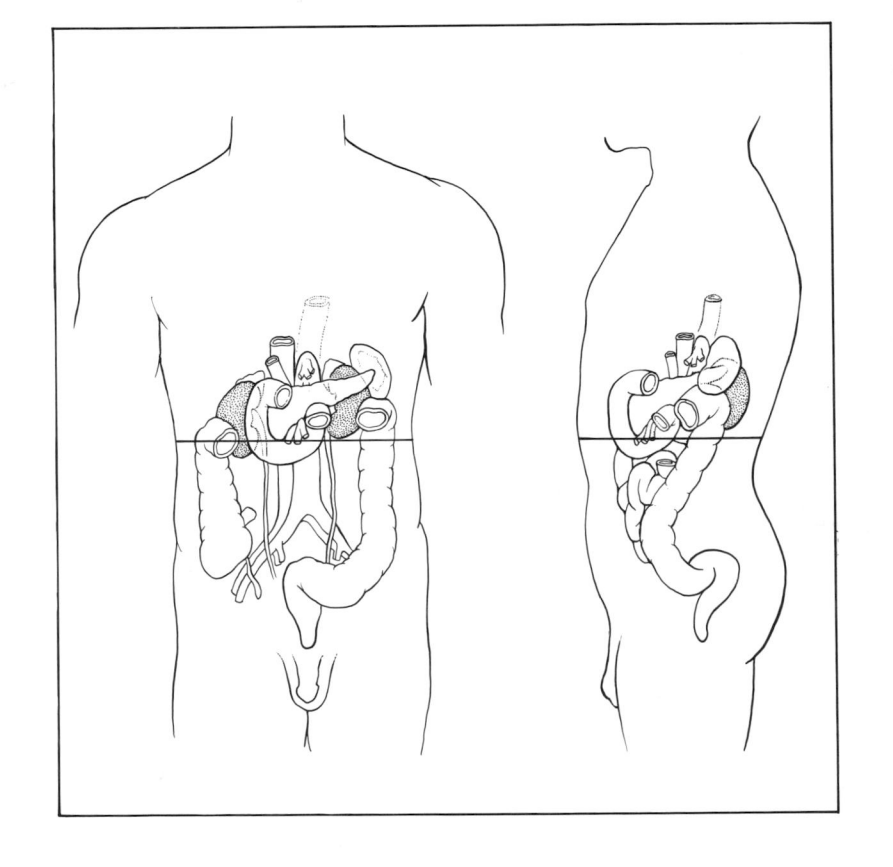

Note

- That **A** is slightly superior to **B**.
- The **right colic flexure** in contact with the surface of the **right kidney** and continuing into the initial segment of the **transverse colon**.
- The **transverse colon**, **pyloric antrum**, and **body of stomach** as the most anterior visceral contents.
- The **ureter** in **A** anterior to the **psoas major muscle** and, in **B**, as it leaves the renal pelvis.
- In **A**, the **left colic flexure** and just posterior to it the **descending colon**.
- In **A**, from right to left, the **inferior vena cava**, **abdominal aorta**, and initial segment of the **fourth part of the duodenum** at the **duodenojejunal junction**.
- In **A**, the termination of the **descending part of the duodenum** and the **third** or transverse **part of the duodenum** passing posterior to the **body of the stomach** and anterior to the **abdominal aorta** and the **inferior vena cava** (*IVC*).
- In **A**, branches of the **superior mesenteric artery** (*SMA*) and tributaries of the **superior mesenteric vein** (*SMV*) lying within the mesentery between the body of the stomach and the transverse part of the duodenum.

Clinical Notes

- The superior mesenteric artery lies close to the anterior aspect of the third part of the duodenum. Hyperextension of the spine can cause the angle between the superior mesenteric artery and the aorta to become even more acute. This in turn causes compression of the third portion of the duodenum. The superior mesenteric artery syndrome is a symptom complex that can result.

References: G 2–28, 2–34, 2–72, 2–73, 2–85, 2–115; RY 293–295

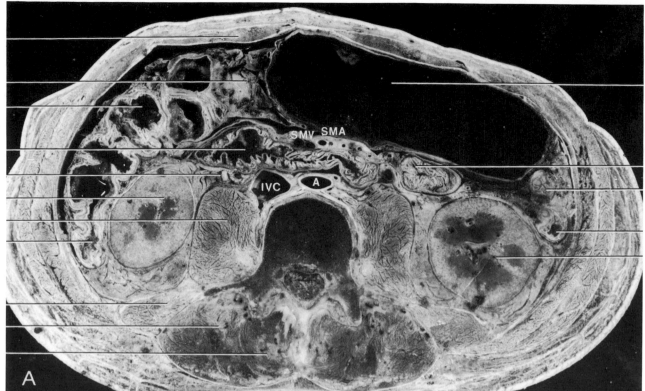

Rectus abdominis

Pyloric antrum

Transverse colon

Third part of duodenum

Ureter

Right kidney

Psoas major

Ascending colon

Quadratus lumborum

Erector spinae

Transversospinalis

SMV SMA

IVC A

Body of stomach

Duodenojejunal junction

Left colic flexure

Descending colon

Left kidney

A

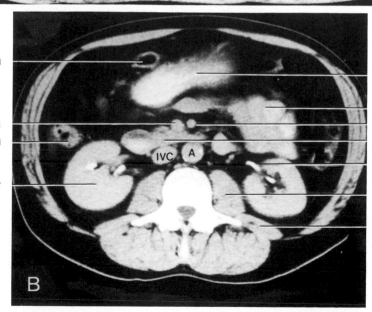

Transverse colon

Superior mesenteric vein

Ascending colon

Right kidney

IVC A

Body of stomach

Jejunum

Superior mesenteric artery

Third part of duodenum

Ureter

Psoas major

Quadratus lumborum

B

A-abdominal aorta   **IVC**-inferior vena cava   **SMA**-superior mesenteric artery   **SMV**-superior mesenteric vein

PLATE 37. Serial transaxial images of abdomen showing gallstones, CT scan, oral and intravenous iodinated contrast

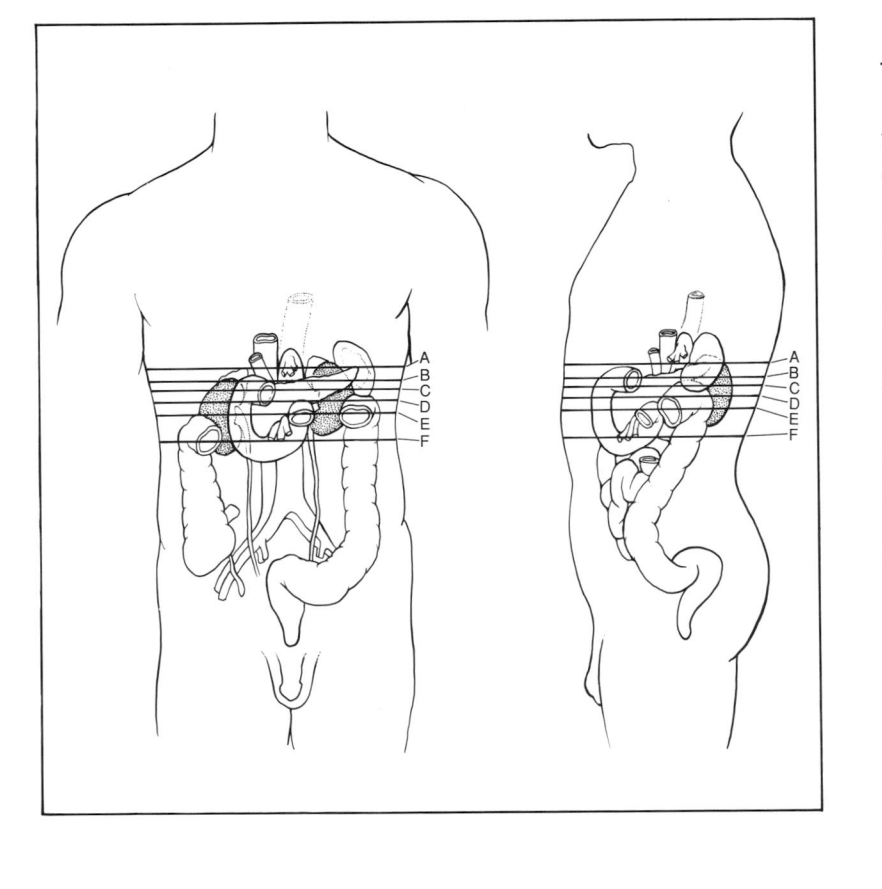

Clinical Notes

- Sequential transaxial images allow one to evaluate the relationships of structures at the various levels. The delineation of masses is critical in the clinical setting, both for differential diagnoses and for determining the possible surgical approach.
- Unopacified bowel is nearly impossible to distinguish from abdominal masses unless contiguous slices are reviewed.
- Review of contiguous sections allows one to evaluate the relationship of lesions to normal structures, such as an abdominal aortic aneurysm to renal artery origins.
- The cavity of the body of the stomach (*sb*) is labeled twice in **B**, **C**, and **D**. The upper label identifies an air density, whereas the lower label identifies contrast medium.
- In evaluating CT scans, the relationship of the superior mesenteric artery hooking anterior to the left renal vein (**C**) is an important one, allowing differentiation from the celiac artery (**B**).
- In this series of CT scans, the gallbladder (*gb*) contains circular calcifications representing at least three gallstones.

References: G 2–28, 2–34, 2–72, 2–73, 2–85, 2–115; RY 293–295

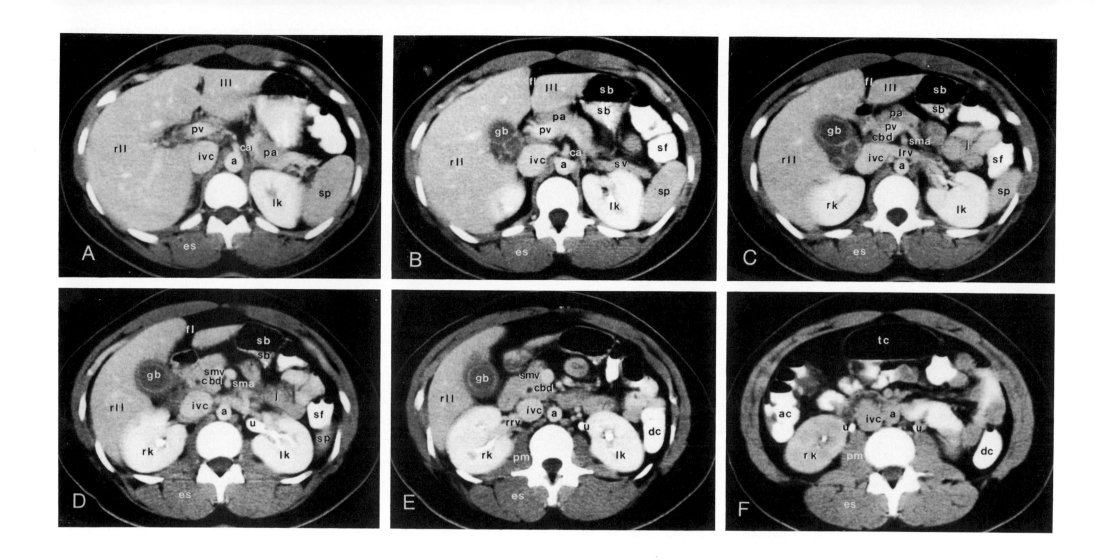

a-abdominal aorta	fl-falciform ligament	lrv-left renal vein	rll-right lobe of liver	sp-spleen
ac-ascending colon	gb-gall bladder	pa-pancreas	rrv-right renal vein	smv-superior mesenteric vein
ca-celiac artery	ivc-inferior vena cava	pm-psoas major	sb-body of stomach	sv-splenic vein
cbd-common bile duct	j-jejunum	pv-portal vein	sf-splenic flexure	tc-transverse colon
dc-descending colon	lk-left kidney	rk-right kidney	sma-superior mesenteric artery	u-ureter
es-erector spinae	lll-left lobe of liver			

PLATE 38. Transaxial section near the abdominopelvic junction, iliac fossa, psoas-iliacus junction, and rectum, T1 MR image

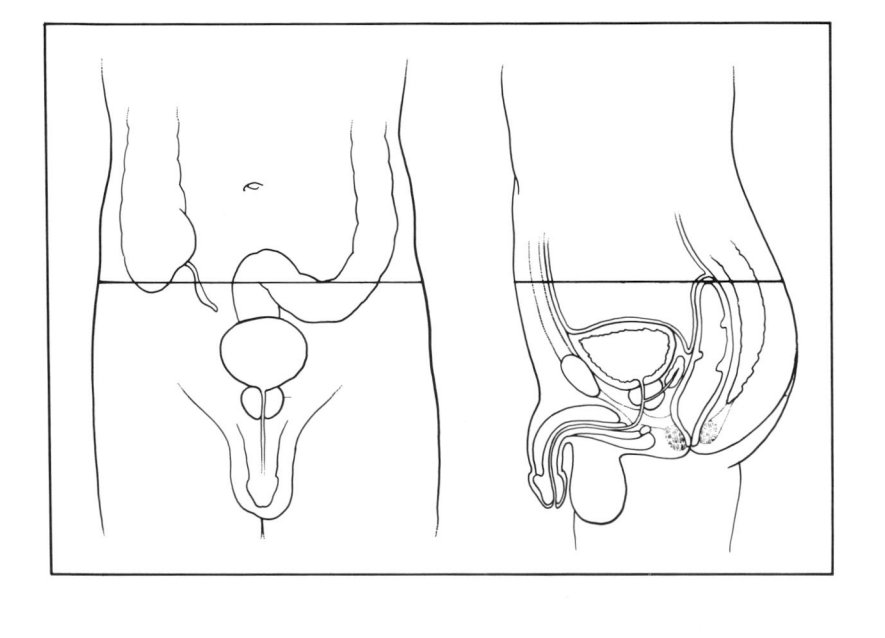

Note

- That **B** is slightly inferior to **A**.
- The **femoral nerve** (*FN*) between the **psoas major** and the **iliacus** muscles.
- Coils of **small bowel**, here primarily made up of **ileum**.
- Posterior and lateral to the ilium, the gluteal muscles: **gluteus maximus**, **gluteus medius**, and **gluteus minimus**.
- In **A**, the **ilium** sectioned on a plane close to the anterior superior iliac spine.
- In **A**, the juxtaposition of the **iliacus** in the iliac fossa and the **psoas major** muscles as they merge to form the iliopsoas muscle.
- In **A**, embedded in the retroperitoneal fascia, alongside the psoas muscle, the **external iliac** and **internal iliac** arteries, and between them the **external iliac vein**.
- In **A**, heading to the **rectum** (*R*) and coursing anterior and medial to the **psoas major** muscle, the **sigmoid colon**.
- In **A**, the continuation of the spinal canal into the **sacral canal** containing the cauda equina.

Clinical Notes

- Adenopathy is commonly seen along the iliac lymph node chains in the region of the main trunk and branches or tributaries of the common iliac artery and vein.

References: G 2–33, 2–34

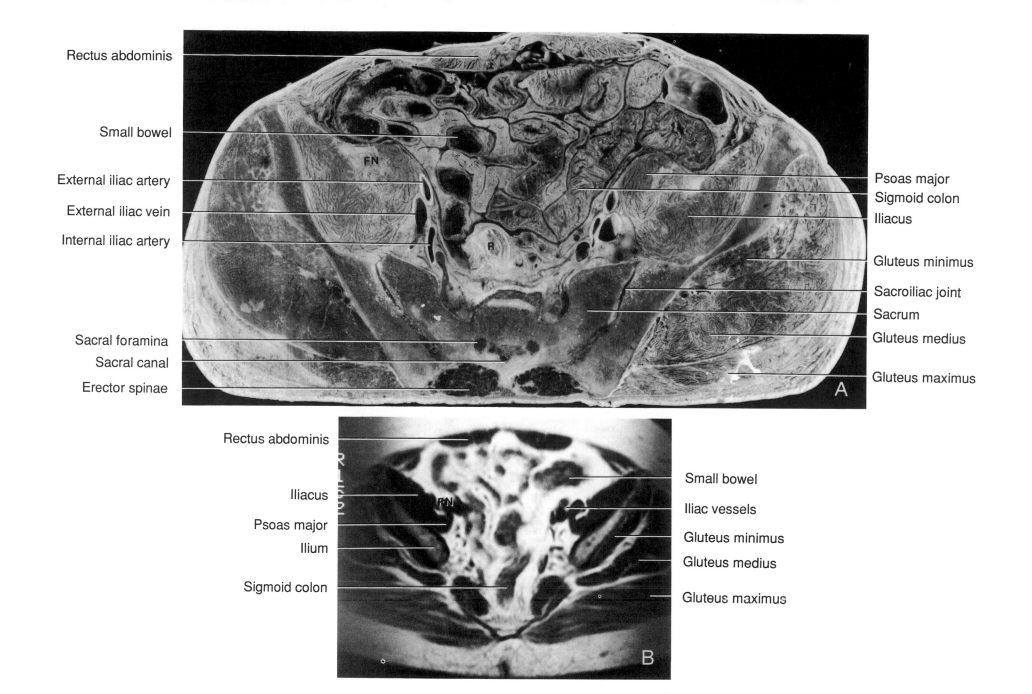

Rectus abdominis

Small bowel

External iliac artery

External iliac vein

Internal iliac artery

Sacral foramina

Sacral canal

Erector spinae

FN

R

Psoas major

Sigmoid colon

Iliacus

Gluteus minimus

Sacroiliac joint

Sacrum

Gluteus medius

Gluteus maximus

A

Rectus abdominis

Iliacus

Psoas major

Ilium

Sigmoid colon

FN

Small bowel

Iliac vessels

Gluteus minimus

Gluteus medius

Gluteus maximus

B

FN-femoral nerve
R-rectum

Section VI. PLATE 38. *Abdominopelvic Junction, Iliac Fossa, Psoas-Iliacus Junction, and Rectum* 77

PLATE 40. Transaxial section, male pelvis minor, through the pubis, seminal vesicles, prostate, and coccyx, T1 MR image

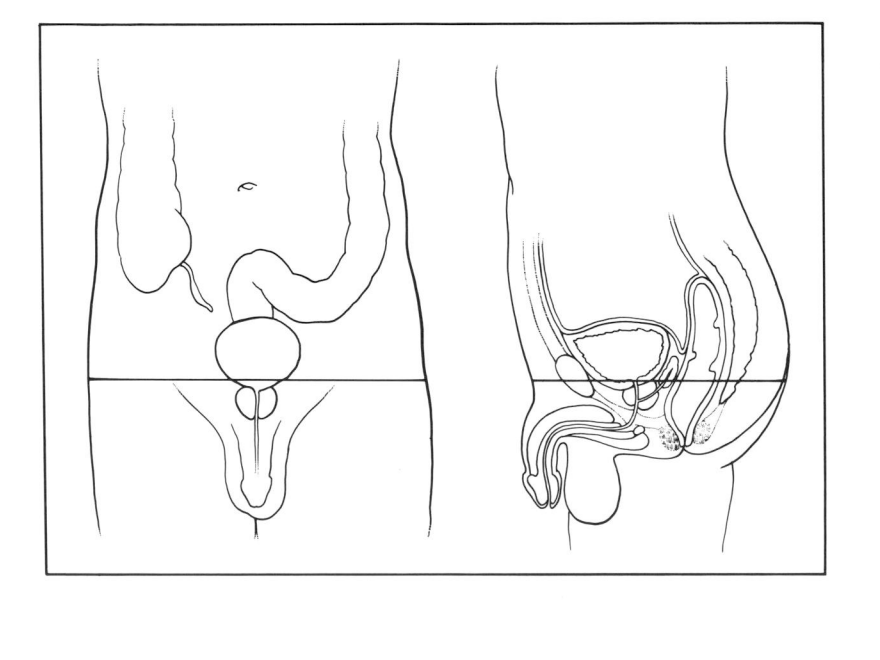

Note

- The **head of the femur** with the **acetabulum** and the **greater trochanter**.
- Posteromedial to the **lesser trochanter** of the femur, the **sciatic nerve** in **A** and in **B** identified as the **region of the sciatic nerve** because the nerve although present is not seen.
- The superior edge of the **prostate gland** close to the neck of the **urinary bladder** and just anterior to the **ampulla of the vas deferens** (*AV*), which itself lies between the **seminal vesicles**.
- In **A**, the **rectum**, lying posterior to the **ampulla of the ductus deferens** (*AV*) and the **seminal vesicles**.
- In **A**, the **femoral nerve** (*FN*), **femoral artery** (*FA*), and **femoral vein** (*FV*) and their position between the **psoas** (*PS*) and **pectineus** (*PEC*) muscles.
- In **A**, the **vas deferens** in the spermatic cord which is seen anterior to the **pectineus muscle** (*PEC*).
- In **A**, the relationship of muscles and vessels surrounding the hip joint.
- In **B**, the **levator ani** muscle surrounding the **rectum**.

Clinical Notes

- At the level of the acetabulum the external iliac artery becomes the femoral artery and is just superior to the site of femoral puncture for injections or blood withdrawals. The close relationship of this artery to the hip joint makes it easy to accidentally enter and contaminate the joint when femoral blood is drawn by needle.
- Periprostatic fat, which surrounds the prostate, and perirectal fat are both loci for tumor infiltration.
- The seminal vesicles are difficult to visualize on MR images.

References: G 3–14, 3–38, 3–39, 3–45, 3–46, 3–47; RY 316 (top)

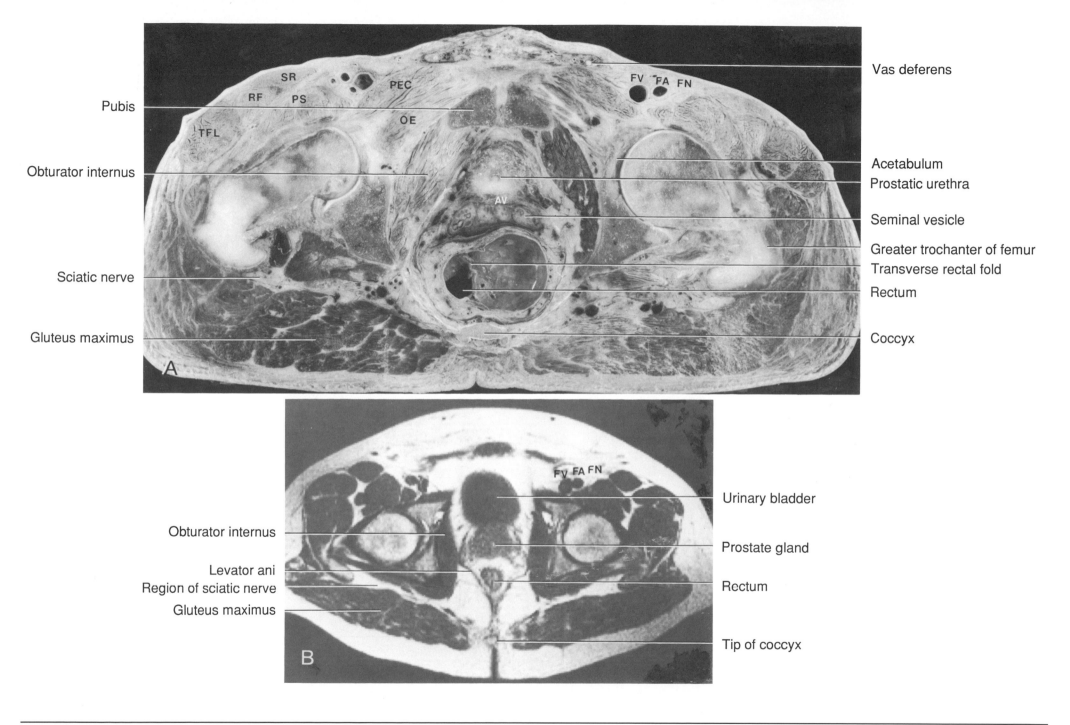

A

Vas deferens

Pubis

SR

RF   PS

PEC

TFL

OE

FV FA FN

Acetabulum

Prostatic urethra

AV

Seminal vesicle

Greater trochanter of femur

Transverse rectal fold

Rectum

Coccyx

Obturator internus

Sciatic nerve

Gluteus maximus

B

FV FA FN

Obturator internus

Levator ani

Region of sciatic nerve

Gluteus maximus

Urinary bladder

Prostate gland

Rectum

Tip of coccyx

AV-ampulla of vas deferens   **FN**-femoral nerve   **OE**-obturator externus   **PS**-iliopsoas   **SR**-sartorius
FA-femoral artery   **FV**-femoral vein   **PEC**-pectineus   **RF**-rectus femoris **TFL**-tensor fasciae latae

PLATE 41. Transverse section, male pelvis minor, level of midprostate, inferior ramus of pubis, T1 MR image

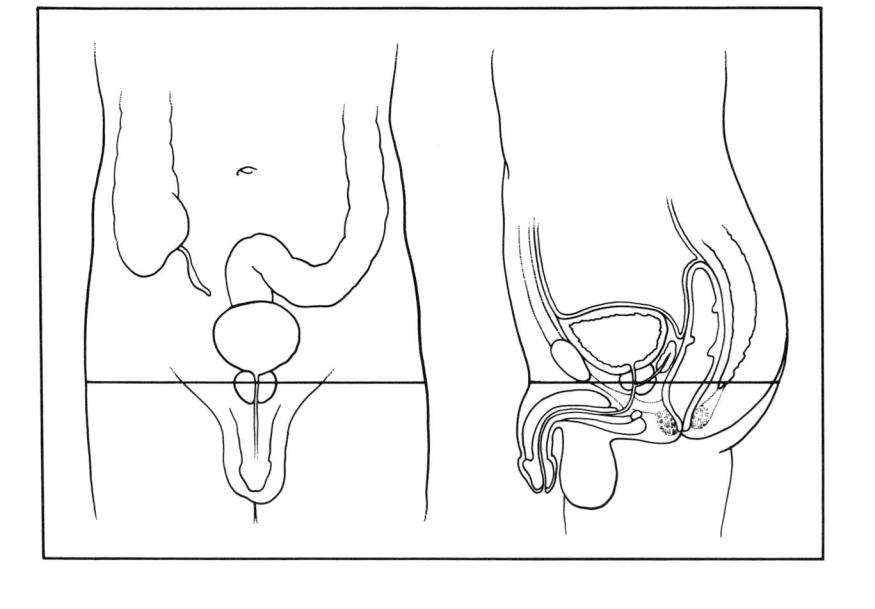

Note

- The **prostate gland** and the **prostatic urethra** lying anterior to the **rectum**.
- The **femoral artery** lying lateral to the **femoral vein** and medial to the **femoral nerve**.
- The **sciatic nerve** between the **ischial tuberosity** and the **lesser trochanter of the femur**.
- On both sides of the **rectum**, the **ischiorectal fossae**, whose copious fat content gives the bright signal seen in **B**.
- In **A**, the slightly biased cut nearer to the level of the top of the **neck of the femur**.
- In **A**, the inferior ramus of the **pubic bone** and, extending laterally from it, the **obturator externus muscle**, anterior to which lie **adductor longus** (*AL*) and **adductor brevis** (*AB*) muscles.

Clinical Notes

- Prostatic cancer often penetrates the capsule and extends into the periprostatic fat. Perirectal fat is also a locus for tumor infiltration.
- The ischiorectal fossae communicate with each other over the anococcygeal ligament. Thus, infection in one fossa may spread to the other.

References: G 3–14, 3–38, 3–39, 3–45, 3–46, 3–47; RY 316 (top)

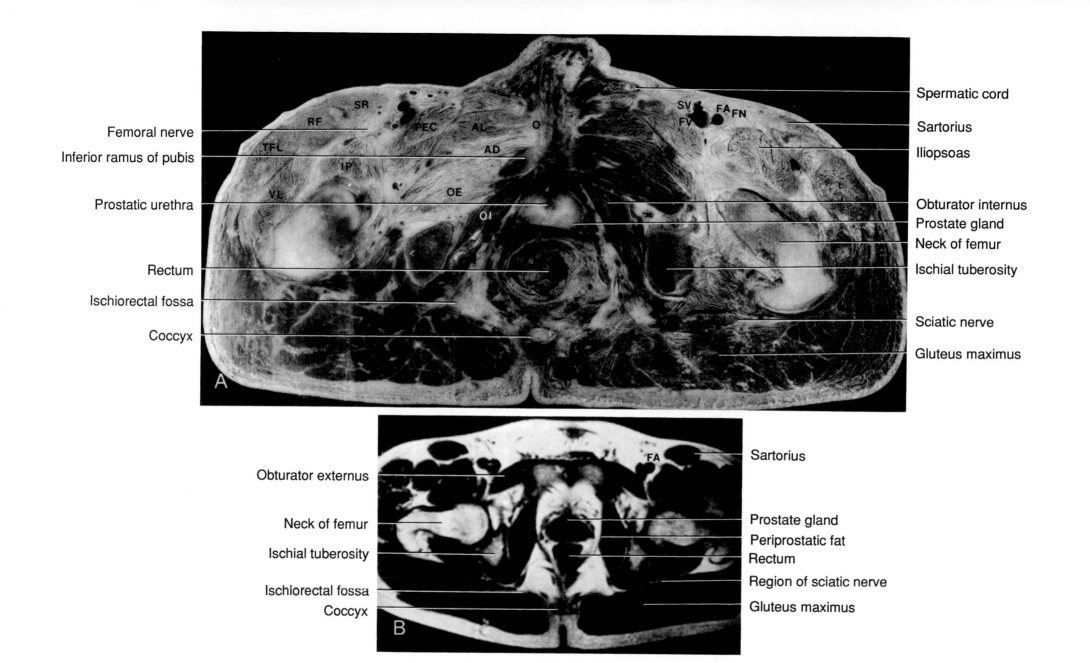

Femoral nerve

Inferior ramus of pubis

Prostatic urethra

Rectum

Ischiorectal fossa

Coccyx

Spermatic cord

Sartorius

Iliopsoas

Obturator internus
Prostate gland
Neck of femur

Ischial tuberosity

Sciatic nerve

Gluteus maximus

Obturator externus

Neck of femur

Ischial tuberosity

Ischiorectal fossa

Coccyx

Sartorius

Prostate gland
Periprostatic fat
Rectum

Region of sciatic nerve

Gluteus maximus

AD-adductor brevis	FN-femoral nerve	OE-obturator externus	RF-rectus femoris	TFL-tensor fasciae latae
AL-adductor longus	FV-femoral vein	OI-obturator internus	SR-sartorius	VL-vastus lateralis
FA-femoral artery	IP-iliopsoas	PEC-pectineus	SV-saphenous vein	

PLATE 42. Transaxial section of male pelvis minor, level of crura of penis, ischial tuberosities, and tip of coccyx, T1 MR image

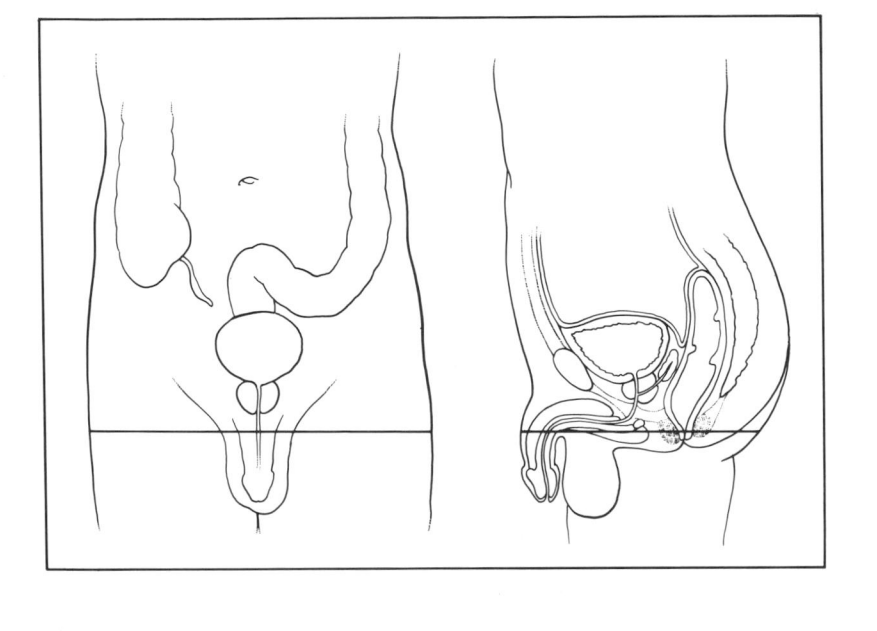

Note

- The **corpus cavernosum** of the penis surrounded by deep penile fascia (Buck's fascia).
- In **A**, the **membranous urethra** at the urogenital diaphragm.
- In **A**, the right **ischial tuberosity** and extending anteriorly from it the ischiopubic ramus, medial to which is the **ischiocavernosus muscle**.
- In **A**, the **femoral artery** between the **femoral vein** and, on its lateral side, the **femoral nerve**.
- In **A**, the **gluteus maximus muscle** and the neurovascular bundle, consisting of the **sciatic nerve**, **inferior gluteal artery**, and **inferior gluteal vein**.

Clinical Notes

- At the level of the coccyx, the sciatic neurovascular bundle can usually be identified on MR images. This is crucial for percutaneous transgluteal drainage of deep pelvic abscesses, because an approach medial to these structures must be taken to avoid damage to the sciatic nerve.
- The pelvis is ideally suited for MR imaging, since intrapelvic organs do not move and there is little motion artifact. Multiplane imaging allows delineation of tumor planes in coronal, sagittal, and other oblique orientations as well as in the standard transaxial planes.
- MR imaging excels in the evaluation of inguinal adenopathy. For example, the regions of the inguinal and femoral canals are seen and, in evaluations of mechanical bowel obstruction of uncertain origin, incidental hernias can usually be diagnosed. Thus, in this slice, if an abdominal mass were seen adjacent to the spermatic cord, it might represent a hernia.

References: G 3–14, 3–17, 3–38, 3–39, 3–45, 3–46, 3–47; RY 316 (top)

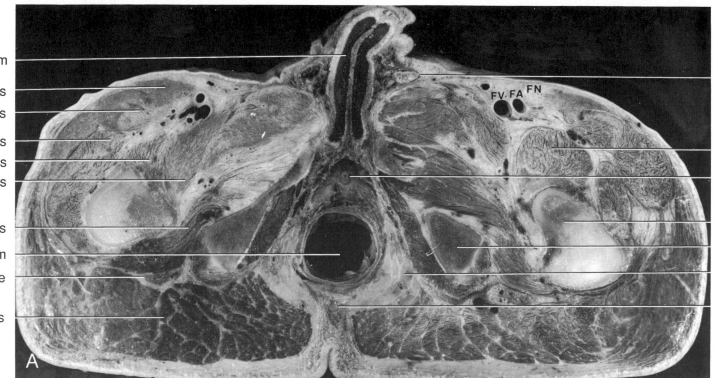

Corpus cavernosum

Sartorius

Rectus femoris

Vastus lateralis
Vastus intermedius
Vastus medialis

Quadratus femoris

Cavity of rectum

Sciatic nerve

Gluteus maximus

Spermatic cord

FV FA FN

Iliopsoas

Membranous urethra

Neck of femur

Ischial tuberosity

Ischiorectal fossa

Tip of coccyx

A

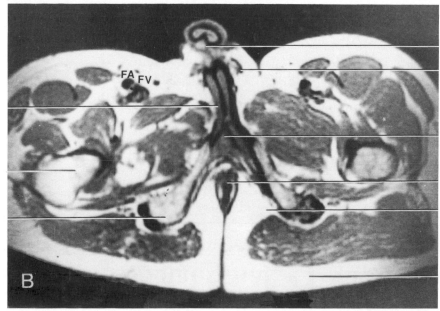

FA FV

Corpus spongiosum

Spermatic cord

Corpus cavernosum

Region of urogenital diaphragm

Neck of femur

Anal canal

Ischial tuberosity

Ischiorectal fossa

Subcutaneous fat

B

FA-femoral artery   **FV**-femoral vein   **FN**-femoral nerve

Section VI. PLATE 42. *Male Pelvis Minor, Crura of Penis, Ischial Tuberosities, and Tip of Coccyx*   85

PLATE 43. Transaxial section of female pelvis major through the cecum, iliac fossa, and spinal canal, T1 MR image

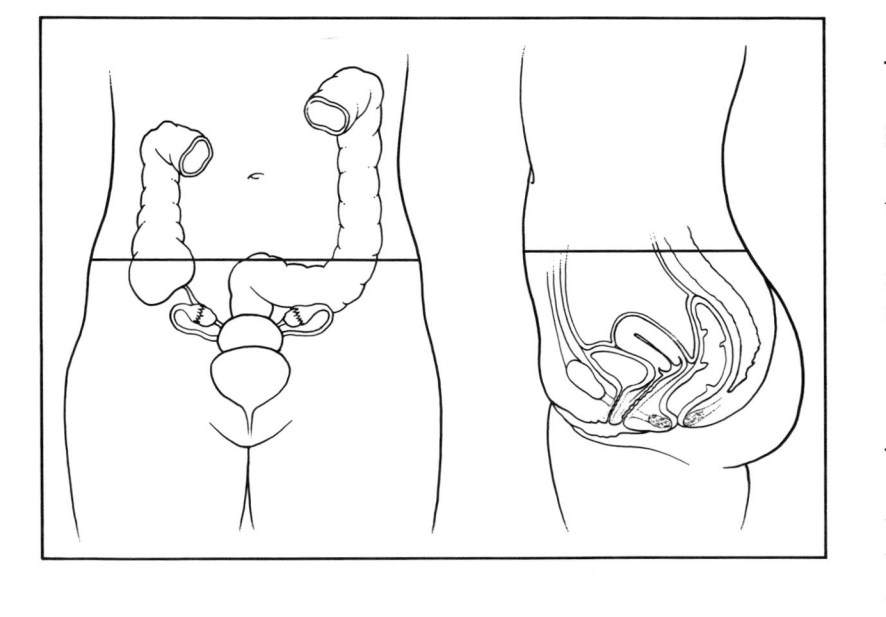

Note

- Embedded in the retroperitoneal fascia and entering the pelvis minor, the **internal iliac artery** (*IIA*), the **internal iliac vein** (*IIV*), and the **external iliac artery** (*EIA*).
- The **mesentery** containing mesenteric arterial branches and venous tributaries and the coils of small bowel, here primarily made up of **ileum**.
- In **A**, posterior and lateral to the ilium, the gluteal muscles—**minimus**, **medius**, and **maximus**—and between minimus and medius the **superior gluteal artery** (*SGA*) and **superior gluteal vein** (*SGV*).
- In **B**, numerous **blood vessels** and **lymph nodes** appear in the fat of the mesentery.

Clinical Notes

- As a result of normal embryological development, rotation of the mesentery causes the direction of drainage into the right lower quadrant. Thus, the cecal region is susceptible to infection. Although abdominal tissue masses can be appreciated on MR imaging, the anatomic resolution of CT scanning is superior, especially when oral contrast material is used to accentuate the bowel.

References: G 2–33, 2–34

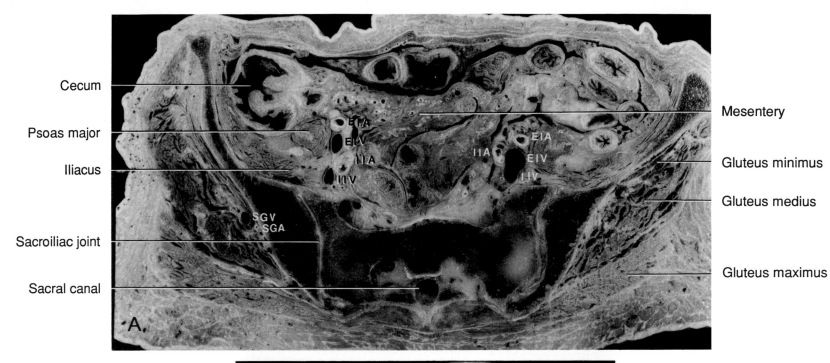

Cecum

Psoas major

Iliacus

Sacroiliac joint

Sacral canal

Mesentery

Gluteus minimus

Gluteus medius

Gluteus maximus

A.

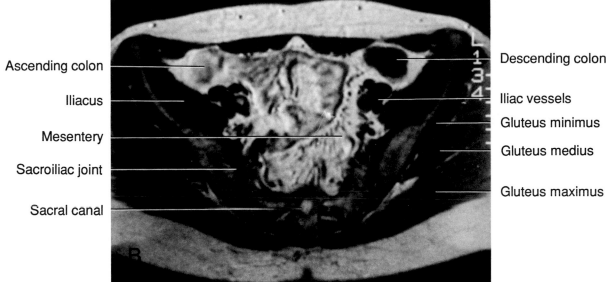

Ascending colon

Iliacus

Mesentery

Sacroiliac joint

Sacral canal

Descending colon

Iliac vessels

Gluteus minimus

Gluteus medius

Gluteus maximus

B.

EIA-external iliac artery　　**IIA**-internal iliac artery　　**SGA**-superior gluteal artery
EIV-external iliac vein　　**IIV**-internal iliac vein　　**SGV**-superior gluteal vein

PLATE 44. Transaxial section of female pelvis minor through the body of the uterus, sigmoid colon, and rectum, T1 MR image

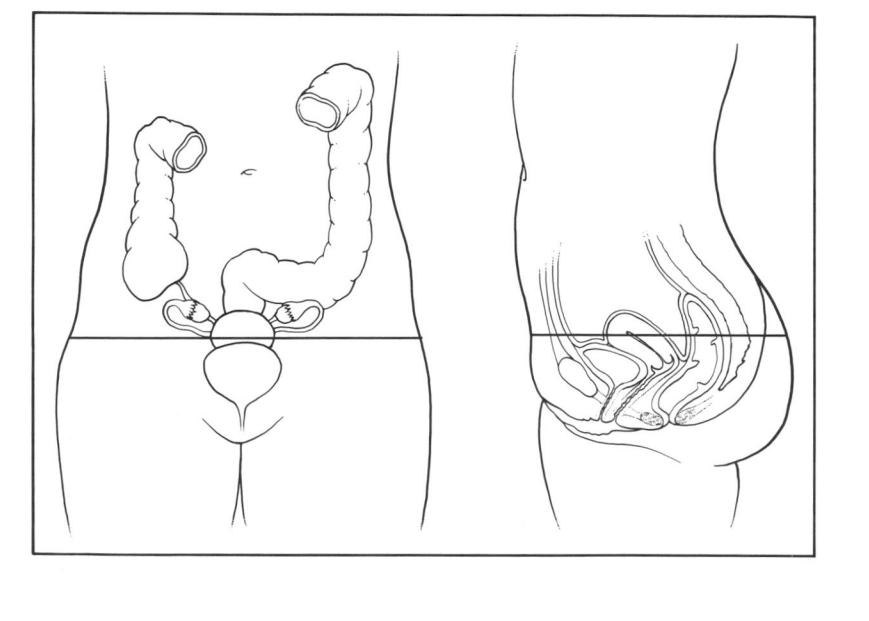

Note

- That while **A** and **B** are at comparable levels, in **B** the **urinary bladder** is filled with urine and hence visible, whereas in **A** it is collapsed and out of the plane of the section.
- The position of the **rectum** relative to the **body of the uterus** and, in **B**, the position of the **bladder** anterior to the **uterus**.
- The relative positions of the **femoral nerve** (*FN*), **femoral artery** (*FA*), and **femoral vein** (*FV*).
- In **A**, the anterior-posterior course of the **sigmoid colon**.
- In **B**, the **uterus**, occupying its normal position relative to the superior surface of the **urinary bladder**.

Clinical Notes

- A most important aspect of staging cervical carcinoma involves the determination of parametrial infiltration. Here, adenopathy around the obturator internus and iliac lymph node chains is well demonstrated in MR images.
- The close approximation of the rectum and uterus make it possible to assess the posterior uterus through a bimanual (simultaneous rectal and vaginal) examination.
- In this example, the patient has an anteverted uterus so that both the fundus (anteriorly) and the cervix (posteriorly) are seen on the same transaxial slice. When slightly enlarged, as in this case, an ovary often contains small benign cysts.

References: G 3–3, 3–11, 3–15; RY 295

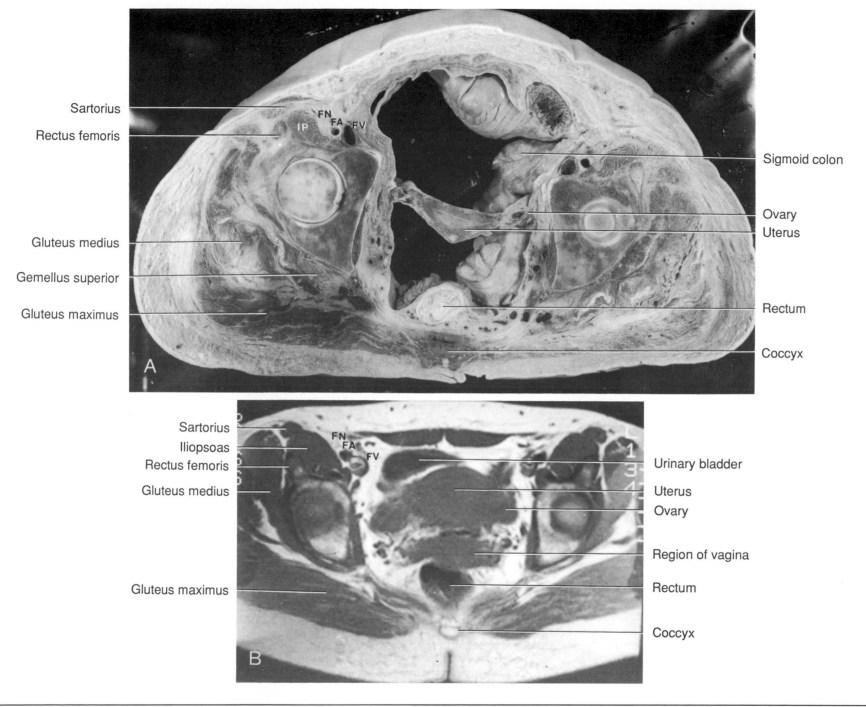

Sartorius

Rectus femoris

FN
IP FA FV

Sigmoid colon

Gluteus medius

Ovary

Uterus

Gemellus superior

Gluteus maximus

Rectum

Coccyx

A

Sartorius

Iliopsoas

FN
FA
FV

Rectus femoris

Gluteus medius

Urinary bladder

Uterus

Ovary

Region of vagina

Gluteus maximus

Rectum

Coccyx

B

FA-femoral artery   **FV**-femoral vein
FN-femoral nerve   **IP**-iliopsoas

PLATE 45. Transaxial section of female pelvis minor through pubis, urinary bladder, and rectum, T1 MR image

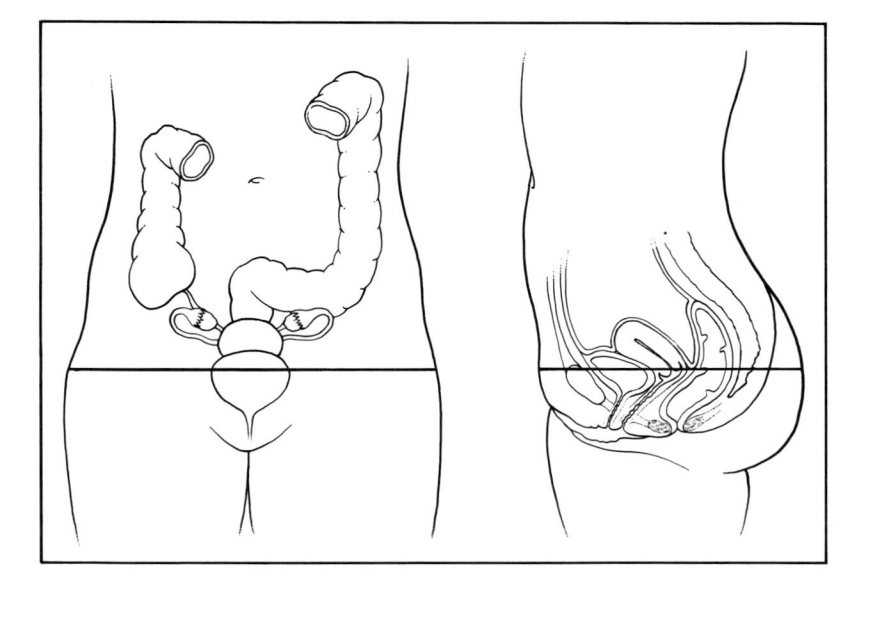

Note

- The important relative positions of the **vagina**, **urinary bladder**, and **rectum**.
- The similarities of muscular and blood vessel structures on this plate to the male pelvis (Plate 40), comparing also the position here of the **round ligament** and that of the **spermatic cord** in Plate 40.
- In **B**, parametrial fat is well defined between the obturator **internus muscle** and the **uterus**.

Clinical Notes

- The degree to which infiltration of the parametrium occurs is an important aspect of staging cervical carcinoma.
- The transaxial view of the femoral heads is part of the MR imaging evaluation of avascular necrosis of the femoral head, which further includes coronal images. This diagnosis is based on evaluation of bone marrow, which is particularly well seen on MR images.

References: G 3-15, 3-35, 3-59, 3-60; RY 328 (lower figure)

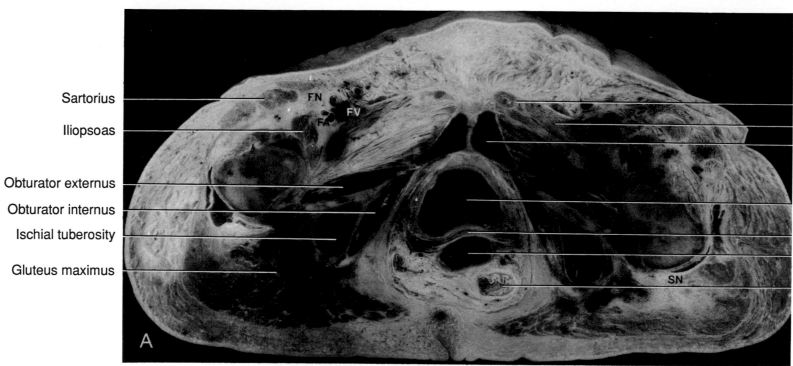

Sartorius

Iliopsoas

Obturator externus

Obturator internus

Ischial tuberosity

Gluteus maximus

FN

FV

FA

SN

A

Round ligament

Pectineus

Pubis

Urinary bladder

Vagina

Rectum

Sigmoid colon

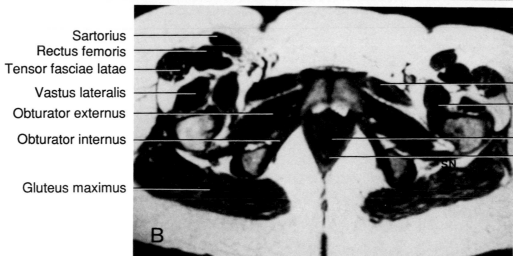

Sartorius
Rectus femoris
Tensor fasciae latae

Vastus lateralis

Obturator externus

Obturator internus

Gluteus maximus

SN

B

Pectineus

Iliopsoas

Region of uterine cervix

Rectum

SN-sciatic nerve
FN-femoral nerve

FA-femoral artery
FV-femoral vein

PLATE 46. Transaxial section of thigh at level of subsartorial canal, quadriceps and sartorius muscles, sciatic nerve, T1 MR image

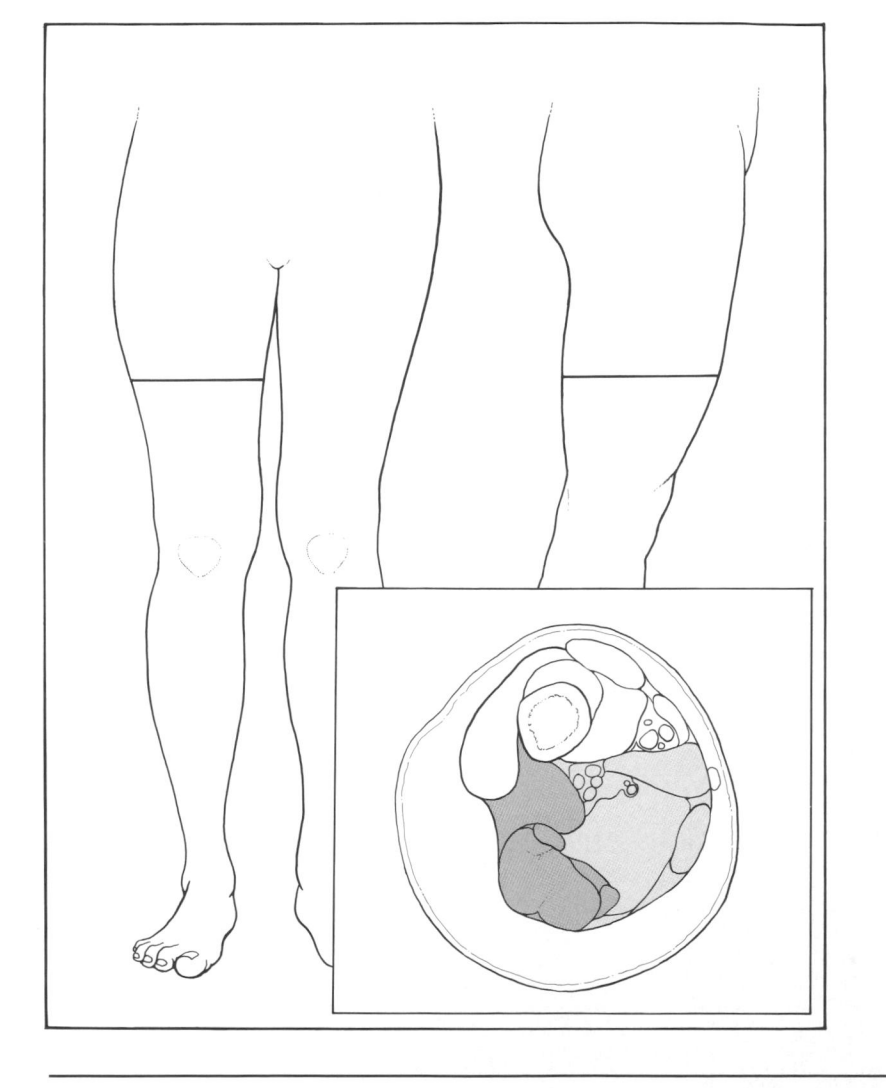

Note

- In the accompanying diagram, the basic compartmentalization of the thigh created by the medial and lateral intermuscular septa and the femur.
- That the anterior musculature, i.e., **rectus femoris**, **vastus medialis**, **vastus lateralis**, and (not labeled) vastus intermedius wrap the femur anteriorly, laterally, and medially.
- The subsartorial canal, whose muscular boundaries are the **adductor longus** posteriorly, **vastus medialis** laterally, and **sartorius** medially.
- The **long saphenous vein** medial to the **adductor longus** muscle embedded in fatty, subcutaneous tissue.
- The **sciatic nerve** as the major nerve component of the posterior compartment.

Clinical Notes

- Since the anterior compartment muscles "wrap around" the femur, it is difficult to palpate the femur in this region.
- MR imaging is currently the best modality for imaging soft tissue masses in the extremities.

References: G 4–5, 4–20, 4–26

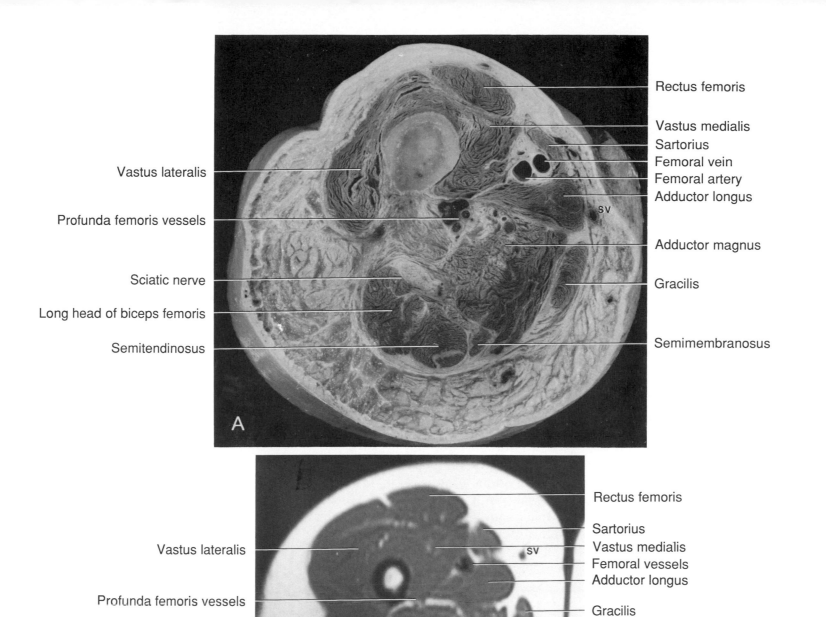

Vastus lateralis

Profunda femoris vessels

Sciatic nerve

Long head of biceps femoris

Semitendinosus

Rectus femoris

Vastus medialis
Sartorius
Femoral vein
Femoral artery
Adductor longus

SV

Adductor magnus

Gracilis

Semimembranosus

A

Vastus lateralis

Profunda femoris vessels

Region of sciatic nerve

Biceps femoris

Semitendinosus

Rectus femoris

Sartorius
Vastus medialis
SV
Femoral vessels
Adductor longus

Gracilis

Adductor magnus

Semimembranosus

B

SV-long saphenous vein

PLATE 47. Transaxial section of the midleg through the tibia, interosseous membrane and fibula, T1 MR image

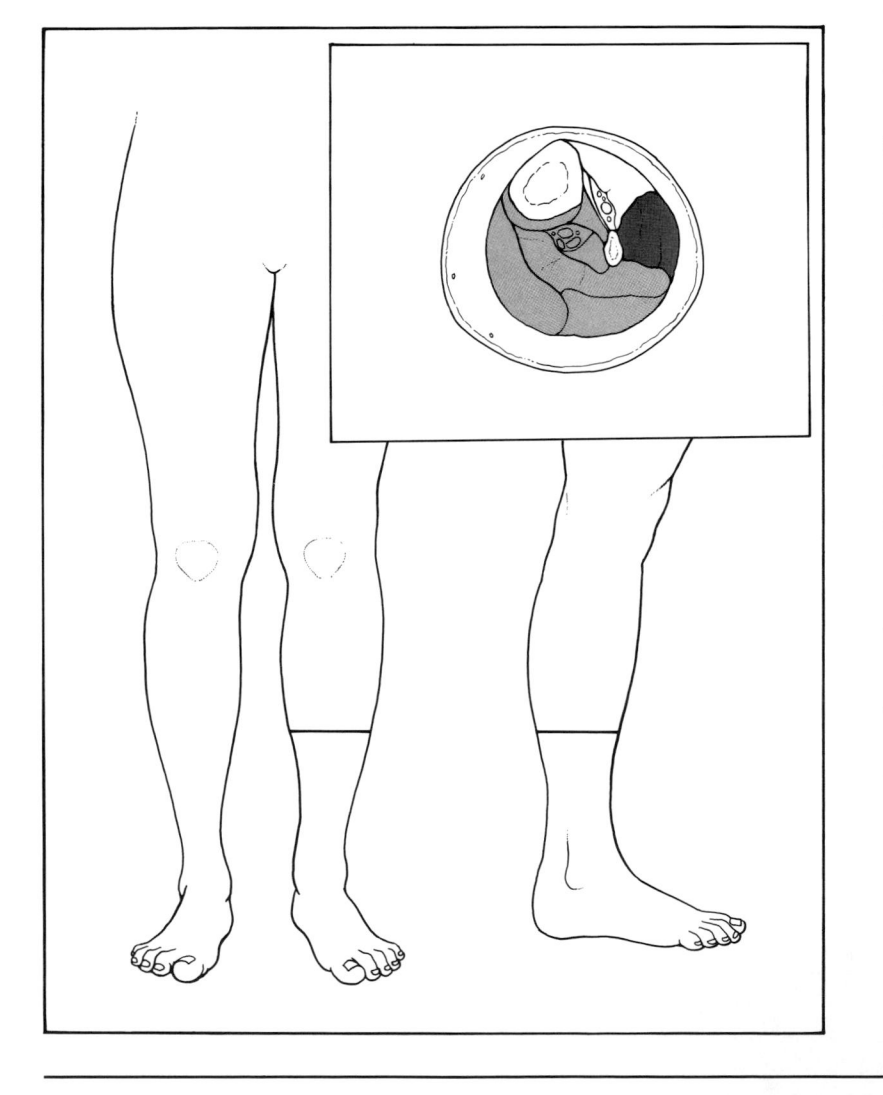

Note

- In the accompanying diagram, the basic compartmentalization of the leg created by the interosseous membrane and the tibia and fibula.
- That the **tibia** (*TI*) on the medial side of the leg is subcutaneous and the **fibula** (*F*) laterally is covered by a thick layer of muscle.
- That **posterior tibial vessels** in **A** and the **region of the posterior tibial artery** lie posterior to the interosseous membrane in the posterior compartment, and that they accompany the tibial nerve, the motor nerve of the posterior compartment of the leg.
- That the **anterior tibial vessels** (artery and vein) accompany the (unlabeled) deep peroneal nerve.
- That the lateral compartment containing the **peroneus longus** and **peroneus brevis** muscles is supplied by here-unseen perforating branches of the peroneal artery from the posterior compartment and receives its nerve supply from the resident nerve, the superficial peroneal.

Clinical Notes

- Focal swelling, within compartments created by fascial planes, may cause ischemia and clinical "compartment syndrome."
- Popliteal cysts adjacent to the lateral head of the gastrocnemius muscle can be seen on MR images, although routine x-ray arthrography and diagnostic ultrasound will also show this pathological condition.

References: G 4–6, 4–7, 4–27

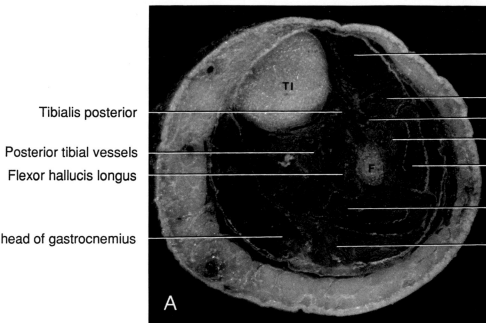

Tibialis anterior

Extensor digitorum longus
Anterior tibial artery
Peroneus brevis
Peroneus longus

Soleus

Lateral head of gastrocnemius

Tibialis posterior

Posterior tibial vessels
Flexor hallucis longus

Medial head of gastrocnemius

A

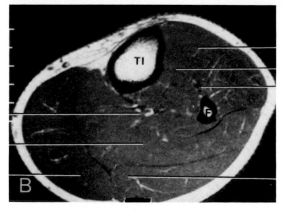

Tibialis anterior
Intermuscular septum
Anterior tibial vessels

Region of posterior tibial vessels

Soleus

Medial head of gastrocnemius

B

Lateral head of gastrocnemius

TI-tibia
F-fibula

Section VII. PLATE 47. *Midleg through Tibia, Interosseous Membrane, and Fibula* 95

PLATE 48.   Transaxial section of the arm, triceps and brachialis muscles, radial nerve, and humerus, T1 MR image

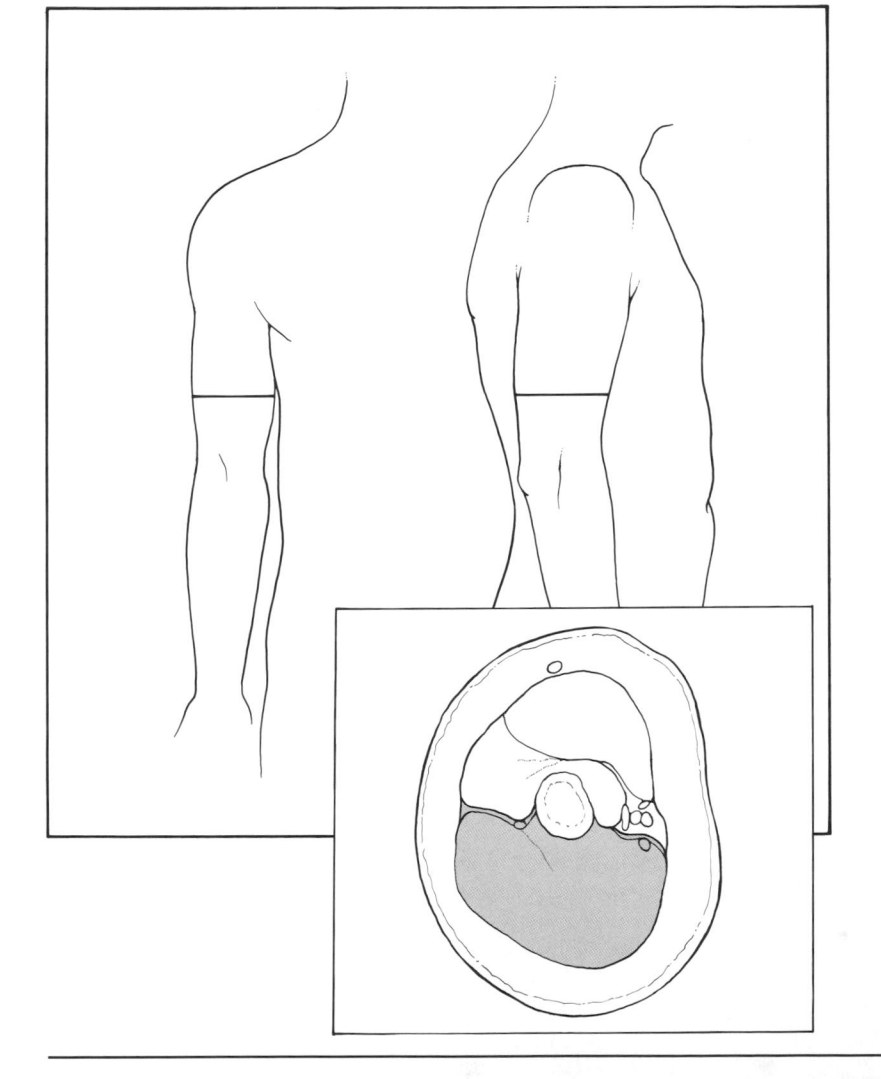

Note

- In the accompanying diagram, the basic compartmentalization of the arm created by the lateral and medial intermuscular septa and the **humerus**.
- The **radial nerve** (*RN*) in the spiral groove in its course from the medial side of the arm to its lateral side, here lying against the **humerus** (*H*) and between the lateral intermuscular septum and the **lateral** and the **medial** heads of the **triceps** muscle.
- In **A**, the region of the **musculocutaneous nerve** lying between the **biceps** and **brachialis** muscles.

Clinical Notes

- The close proximity of the radial nerve to bone makes it vulnerable to injury in fractures of the shaft of the humerus.

References: G 6–39, 6–40B, 6–41

Biceps brachii

Lateral head of triceps

Brachialis

Medial head of triceps

Long head of triceps

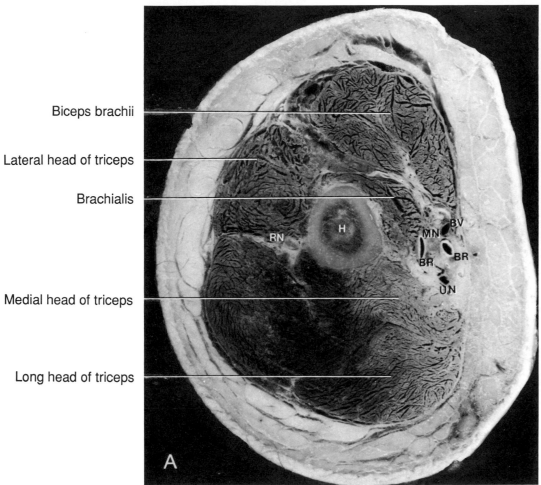

Biceps brachii

Lateral head of triceps

Region of radial nerve

Region of brachial artery

Long head of triceps

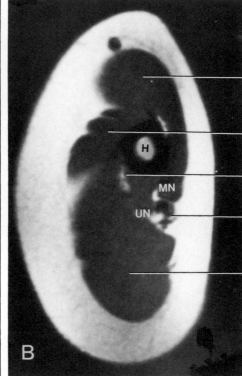

BV-basilic vein   **MN**-median nerve   **RN**-radial nerve
H-humerus   **UN**-ulnar nerve   **BR**-brachial artery

PLATE 49. Transaxial section of the forearm through the brachioradialis tendon, extensor digitorum muscle, and interosseous membrane, T1 MR image

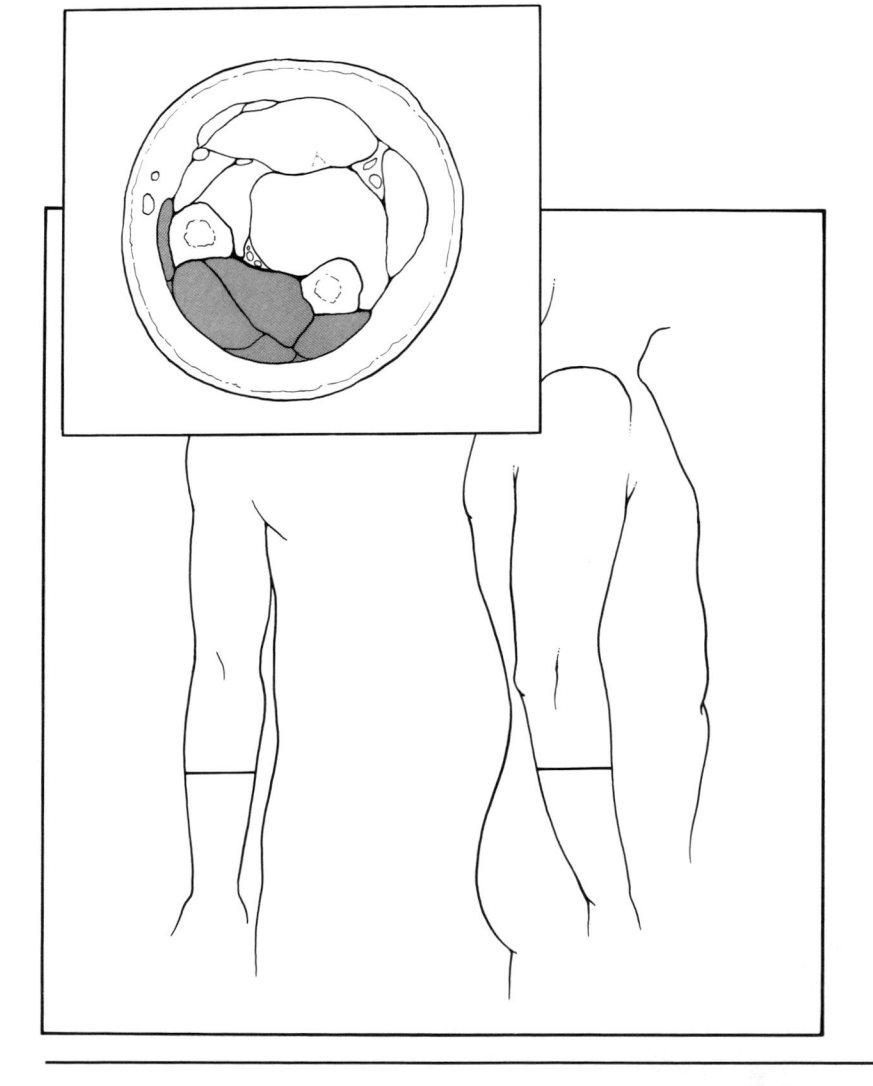

Note

- In the accompanying diagram, the basic compartmentalization of the forearm created by the **interosseous membrane** and **radius** and **ulna**.
- The positions of anterior compartment nerves relative to surrounding muscles, the **median nerve** deep to the **flexor digitorum superficialis**, and the **ulnar nerve** under cover of the **flexor carpi ulnaris**.
- That branches of the posterior interosseous nerve (not seen) lie in the **posterior compartment** behind the interosseous membrane, anterior to which lie the **anterior interosseous nerve** and the **anterior interosseous artery**.

Clinical Notes

- Within the neurovascular bundles flow phenomena can result in varied appearances of blood vessels. In this example, the higher signal (*bright white*) may represent slower flow within the vein of the radial neurovascular bundle.

References: G 6–66, 6–68, 6–69, 6–70, 6–71

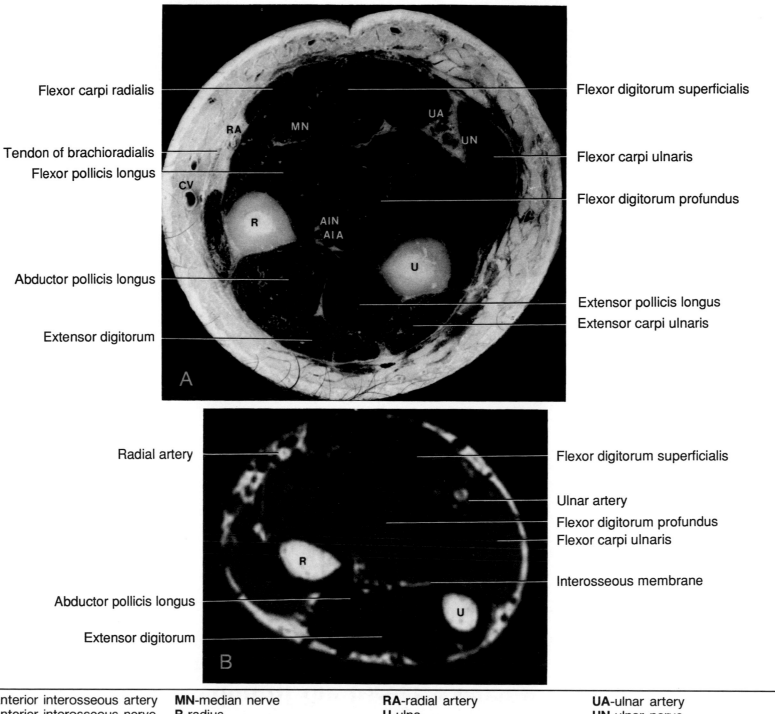

Flexor carpi radialis

Tendon of brachioradialis
Flexor pollicis longus

Abductor pollicis longus

Extensor digitorum

Flexor digitorum superficialis

Flexor carpi ulnaris

Flexor digitorum profundus

Extensor pollicis longus
Extensor carpi ulnaris

Radial artery

Abductor pollicis longus

Extensor digitorum

Flexor digitorum superficialis

Ulnar artery

Flexor digitorum profundus
Flexor carpi ulnaris

Interosseous membrane

AIA-anterior interosseous artery   **MN**-median nerve   **RA**-radial artery   **UA**-ulnar artery
AIN-anterior interosseous nerve   **R**-radius   **U**-ulna   **UN**-ulnar nerve
CV-cephalic vein

PLATE 50. Transaxial section of the hand through the middle palm, metacarpal bones, and adductor pollicis muscle, T1 MR image

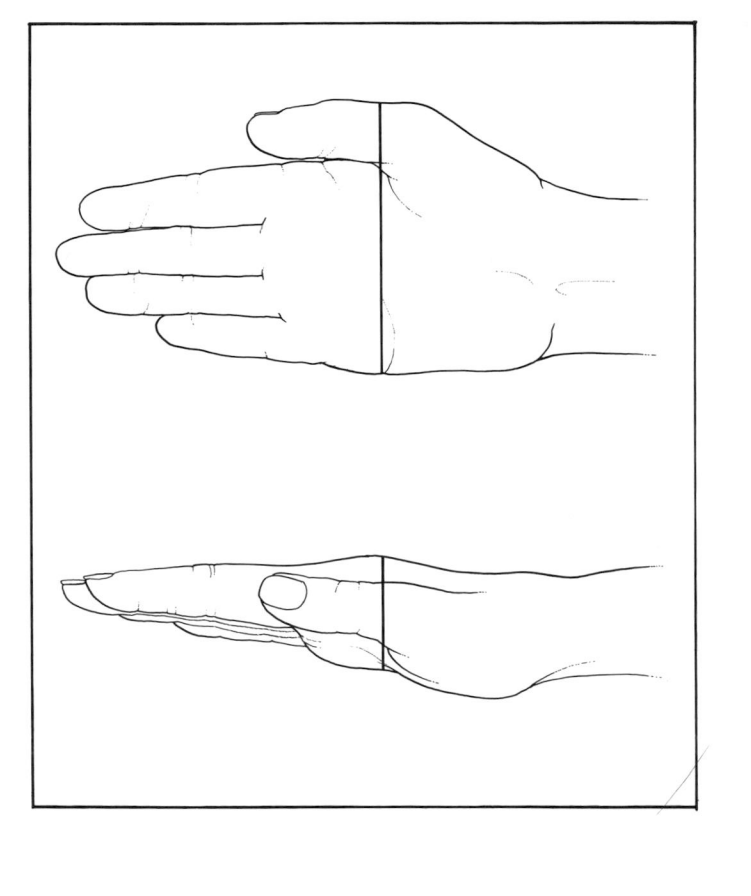

Note

• The hand sectioned at midpalm. In **B**, in the sectioned metacarpal bones, the black signal resembling rings arising from the low signal of cortical bone versus the lighter signal of marrow.

Clinical Notes

• The extent of tumor in the muscle planes of the hand and wrist can best be evaluated by MR imaging.
• Developments in local or surface coil technology continue to improve detail in extremity imaging.
• Small ganglion cysts, often the source of unexplained soft tissue pain, can also be diagnosed, especially on T2-weighted images.
• Unexplained hand pain of possible osseous origin is usually evaluated initially by radionuclide bone imaging.

References: G 6–73, 6–76, 6–84

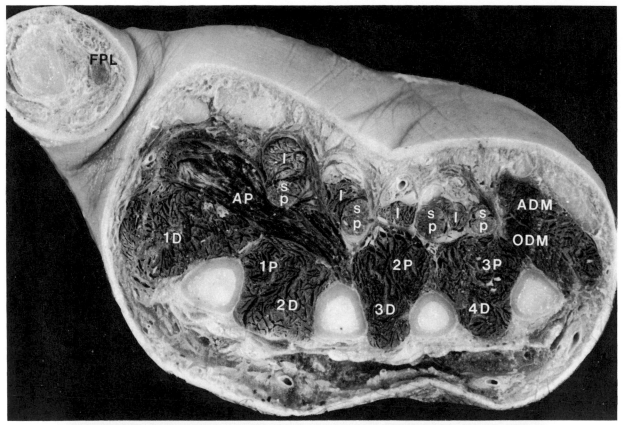

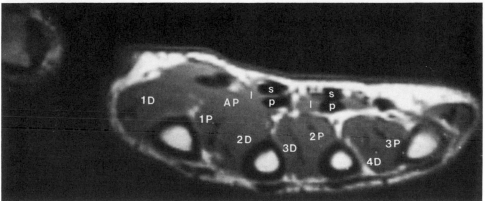

ADM-abductor digiti minimi
AP-adductor pollicis
FPL-flexor pollicis longus
I-lumbrical
ODM-opponens digiti minimi

p-tendons of flexor digitorum
   profundus
s-tendons of flexor digitorum
   superficialis

1P-3P-first through third palmar
   interossei
1D-4D-first through fourth dor-
   sal interossei

Index